SPORT FOR LIFE

STRENGTH TRAINING

Beginners, Bodybuilders, and Athletes

Philip E. Allsen

Brigham Young University

Charles B. Corbin/Philip E. Allsen, Series Editors

Scott, Foresman and Company
Glenview, Illinois   London

SPORT FOR LIFE

BOWLING Joyce M. Harrison *Brigham Young University* Ron Maxey

CYCLING Lee N. Burkett Paul W. Darst *Arizona State University*

JOGGING David E. Corbin *The University of Nebraska at Omaha*

RACQUETBALL Robert P. Pangrazi *Arizona State University*

STRENGTH TRAINING Philip E. Allsen *Brigham Young University*

Charles B. Corbin/Philip E. Allsen, Series Editors

Cover photograph by Robert Drea

Library of Congress Cataloging-in-Publication Data

Allsen, Philip E.
    Strength training.

    (Sport for life)
    Bibliography: p.
    Includes index.
    1. Weight lifting.   2. Physical education and
training.   3. Bodybuilding.   I. Title.   II. Series:
Sport for life series.
GV546.A44   1987   796.4'1   86-26070

ISBN 0-673-18170-7

 2 3 4 5 6 7-KPF-91 90 89 88 87

Foreword

We are calling this series SPORT FOR LIFE because we believe a sports skills series should be more than just a presentation of the "rules of the game." A popular sport or activity should be presented in a way that encourages understanding through direct experience, improvement through prompt correction, and enjoyment through proper mental attitude.

Over the years, each SPORT FOR LIFE author has instructed thousands of people in their selected activity. We are delighted these "master teachers" have agreed to put down in writing the concepts and procedures they have developed successfully in teaching a skill.

The books in the SPORT FOR LIFE Series present other unique features as appropriate to the featured sport or activity.

The Sport Experience: This is a learning activity that explains and teaches a technique or specific rule. Whether it requires the reader to experience selecting a specific bicycle, stroking a backhand in tennis, or choosing an approach to use in bowling it carries the learner right to the heart of the game or activity at a pace matching his or her own progress. The Sport Experience is identified throughout the book with its own special typographical design.

The Error Corrector: The SPORT FOR LIFE authors have taken specific skills and listed some of the common errors encountered by participants; at the same time they have listed the methods to be utilized to correct these errors. The Error Corrector can be compared to a road map as it provides checkpoints toward skillful performance of a sport or activity.

The Mental Game: Understanding the mental game can remove many of the obstacles to success. The authors have devised techniques to aid the reader in planning playing strategy and in learning how to cope with the stress of competition. It is just as important to know how to remove mental errors as it is to deal with the physical ones.

The editors and authors of SPORT FOR LIFE trust that their approach and enthusiasm will have a lasting effect on each reader and will help promote a lifetime of health and happiness, physically and psychologically, for a sport well played or an activity well performed.

Charles B. Corbin/Philip E. Allsen

About the Author and Editors

Philip E. Allsen.   Dr. Allsen is also co-editor of this book and information about him is found below.

Charles B. Corbin.   Dr. Corbin is Professor of Physical Education at Arizona State University. A widely known expert on fitness and health, he is author or co-author of 27 books on those topics addressed to students ranging from the elementary school through college. In August 1986 he was given the "Better Health and Living Award" by that magazine as one of 10 Americans who have made the difference in influencing others in the areas of health and fitness. He is a 1982 recipient of the National Honor Award from the American Alliance for Health, Physical Education, Recreation and Dance and is a fellow in the American Academy of Physical Education.

Philip E. Allsen.   Dr. Allsen is Professor of Physical Education and Director of the Fitness for Life Program at Brigham Young University in Provo, Utah. Widely known for his expertise in physical fitness, sports medicine, and athletic training, Dr. Allsen, a prolific writer, has authored more than 75 articles and written 16 books covering the topics of strength and physical fitness. The "Fitness for Life" program, which Dr. Allsen developed at Brigham Young University, now serves approximately 7,000 students at the institution each year and has been adopted by more than 400 schools in the United States. He is a member of the American College of Sports Medicine, the American Alliance of Health, Physical Education, Recreation and Dance, and the National Collegiate Physical Education Association.

Preface

Anyone who is interested in increasing their performance, whether in athletics or any other aspect of life, can do so by increasing body strength. *Strength Training: Beginners, Bodybuilders, and Athletes* has been written to present strength development programs for beginning strength trainers, for those who wish to use strength to improve their athletic ability, and for those interested in becoming serious bodybuilders.

The author has had the opportunity to supervise strength training programs for thousands of people. They have ranged from individuals who have never participated in any type of strength program to elite athletes who are competing on the professional level. In addition, physique athletes have been trained who have gone on to win national contests in bodybuilding.

The first two chapters of this book give a scientific background on the physiological and anatomical changes brought about by engaging in a strength development program. The basic concepts necessary to understand strength programs are also presented in these two chapters.

The last chapters deal with the actual designing of the specific strength programs that the reader may wish to engage in. To help in developing a total and comprehensive training program, there is a presentation of many different exercises for each of the specific muscle groups. This section allows one to select a variety of exercises to strengthen the various body parts. Each exercise is illustrated by pictures that demonstrate the correct body position and technique to utilize. The pictures are accompanied by explanations of the action and precautions to use. By applying these concepts, it is easy to design programs that are safe and efficient.

It is the considered judgment of the author that strength training is important for everyone and that this type of training can add a dimension to life that ensures greater productivity and enjoyment of self-concept that is positive and beneficial.

Contents

Why Train for Strength?

So often when the word *strength* enters into a conversation, people think primarily of men with bulging muscles or NFL football players crashing into one another on the field of battle. The question is then asked why the normal individual living an everyday life would give any serious consideration to engaging in a strength training program. It has been the author's experience to have people make statements such as, "Why, I am only a homemaker" or "What good will increased strength do for me in my business as a computer programmer?"

To answer these questions and dispel some of the misconceptions surrounding the topic of strength, we will spend some time explaining what strength is and why strength can give everyone an advantage in participating in the activities of daily life.

STRENGTH AND ITS ADVANTAGES

Strength is defined as the ability to exert force against resistance. Force is the basis of all motion, and when we examine the world we live in we can easily observe that it is a world of motion. Strength then becomes an important aspect in performing the tasks of daily living, such as lifting, walking, running, doing housework, and engaging in recreational tasks.

Another aspect of movement is *power*. Power is defined in terms of the rate at which energy can be released, or the rate of doing work. The formula for power is:

$$\text{Power} = \frac{\text{force} \times \text{distance}}{\text{time}}$$

Distance divided by time equals speed, and thus the two factors in power are force, or strength, and speed. To affect power, a training program must affect either strength or speed or, if possible, both of these factors at the same time. Of these two variables, it is much more difficult to bring about changes in speed than in strength. The major key to developing increased power is thus the change that a training program can bring about on the development of strength.

As you can see, power becomes one of the keys to a more productive life. It has been said that it is not time that is important but what takes place in time that is the difference between success and failure. By increasing your power output you can accomplish more work in a shorter period of time.

Let us use a practical example of mowing the lawn. If you increase your strength and bring about a greater power output, the work of mowing the lawn can be accomplished much more quickly. A friend of the author gave the following reason for participating in a strength program: "I can finish my yardwork in a short period of time, and this allows me to get on the golf course where I can apply force to the golf ball with a great amount of joy!"

The past few years have seen some remarkable performances in athletic achievement. Athletes are jumping further and higher, runners are breaking records in most of the running events, and swimming records are broken in nearly every large swimming meet.

Physiologically, the body has been operating the same way for a long while, so there must be a reason why the human body is breaking athletic records that were thought to be impossible to change. When we examine the training procedures these record-breaking athletes engage in, we find that one of the greatest causes of improvement is the proper use of a strength training program.

If strength is the ability to exert force and force is a tendency to cause motion, then strength is important not only to the athlete but to all individuals in everyday life. If more work can be accomplished in a shorter period of time, a person is more powerful. If all else remains equal, an increase in strength will contribute to an improvement in the performance of the human body.

Other reasons for engaging in strength training are that it makes you feel better and look better. A person does not have to be a so-called bodybuilder to value the effect on the self-concept of an attractive body. The author conducted a survey of the men and women engaged in a series of strength development classes, and over 80 percent responded that the major reason for taking the class was that they wished "to look better."

Since many people express a desire to look better, it is necessary to discuss body composition. The human body is composed of materials which are referred to as *lean body mass* and *fat mass*. Lean body mass is made up primarily of muscle tissue, bone, and fluids, and fat mass is the fat that the body stores. One of the problems in our society is that many people have an excess amount of body fat, and this leads to the problems of obesity. It is estimated that by the age of fifty, almost 50 percent of the people in the United States are approaching obesity, or over-fatness.

The relationship between the amount of muscle mass in the body and excess body fat is often overlooked. The amount and size of muscle decrease in many people as they get older because of a lack of a strength training stimulus. As the muscle mass decreases, the person uses less energy even at rest, and a greater percentage of the body weight becomes fat. Fat tissue does not burn nearly as many calories at rest as muscle tissue, and thus the individual continues to gain body fat. In other words, many people become fat because they are using fewer calories as a result of the loss of muscle mass caused by a lack of activity. Since people spend more time in sitting than in any other activity, the average American becomes over-fat as he or she grows older.

Ancel Keys, a researcher in weight control, showed that the decrease in caloric expenditure in different age groups at rest was related to the change in muscle mass rather than to age. For example, at age sixty a person will use approximately fifteen calories less per hour than a person who is twenty-six years of age. Over a twenty-four-hour period this would be a total of 360 unused calories per day. If that person desires to have the same eating habits but not put on fat, it will be necessary to walk approximately six miles each day to expend the 360 calories, since the energy used in walking one mile is about sixty calories. The sixty-year-old individual, therefore, must increase activity, decrease caloric intake, or else put on more fat.

A person can help eliminate the problem of over-fatness by using a strength development program to maintain the muscle mass so that there won't be a decrease in caloric expenditure at rest. Thus a person won't have to exercise so extensively to combat obesity. The body will continue to use more calories if the muscle mass is maintained throughout life.

A misconception that many times arises in regard to strength development is that a strength training program will cause "muscle-boundness," or a loss of flexibility. There have been many scientific studies conducted which refute this myth and indicate that the opposite is true, that engaging in a strength program correctly will actually bring about an improvement in flexibility. One study conducted at the

1972 Olympic Games tested the flexibility of the competing athletes, and it was found that the most flexible athletes were the gymnasts, swimmers, and weight-lifters.

The key to maintaining good flexibility is to take the body parts through a full range of motion, and this can be accomplished by engaging in a proper strength development program. By using correct techniques, you will develop strength throughout the entire range of movement of the body musculature.

The ability of the body to resist the stresses that can result from an injury can be increased by obtaining a greater amount of strength. This is quite obvious to the athletic world, and there are statistics that indicate that athletic injuries, such as in football, are reduced when teams engage in a strength development program. The fatigue of sports participation combats the body's ability to withstand the disruption of movement, but with an increase in strength, the athlete is more powerful and thus retains the ability to perform in the later stages of the contest.

This same advantage is important in performing everyday tasks, such as lifting or carrying objects.

When we examine all the ways strength can contribute to the overall efficiency of the human body, it becomes obvious that a strength development program should be a lifetime process.

WOMEN AND STRENGTH TRAINING

In some instances when strength training is being considered, women become concerned that strength exercises will make them less feminine. There is a fear that training will produce large, unsightly, bulging muscles. In the past few years, research has disputed this myth that has grown up. Women have the same muscle properties as men, but because of endocrinological differences, they respond to a training stimulus in different ways. Before puberty, there is little difference between the muscular size and strength of boys and girls, but with the onset of puberty, testosterone from the testes of the male and estrogen from the ovaries of the female begin to enter the bloodstream and trigger the development of the appropriate secondary sexual characteristics. The result is that men now develop a greater quantity of muscle tissue and will also respond with a greater gain of muscle mass when they engage in a strength program.

In most cases a woman will not get large gains in muscle mass when training, but she will obtain increased strength which will now enable her to better perform daily activities. The cross-section of a muscle cell can increase as much as 30 percent in diameter without measurable growth in the girth of a body limb, so the woman does not have any worry about increased body size. There is no physiological reason for a woman not to engage in a strength training program.

Since a woman has the same general musculature as a man, and her needs are identical to those of the man, there is no need to suggest different training programs on the basis of sex. Both women and men can experience the same general benefits; it is only the degree of gain in muscle tissue that will differ.

OVER FORTY

The question is sometimes asked if older people, that is, people over the age of forty, should engage in strength training. The answer is that all the advantages of increased strength listed in this chapter hold true for any age.

The author has conducted research to compare the rate of strength gains in men and women of various ages. The results show that the rate of strength gain is similar for all age groups.

Our society has tended to be youth oriented to the neglect of its older citizens. If you are an individual who falls into the older age categories, you can rest assured that engaging in a proper strength development program can not only increase your strength but also increase the overall performance of your body.

CONCLUSION

When you make the decision to start a strength program, it indicates that you have started a new lifestyle. It is important to point out that strength is reversible and will decline if you do not continue to obtain a strength stimulus for your entire life.

Principles and Programs

The exact physiological cause of increased strength is not known. Increased strength may be due to changes brought about in the muscular, skeletal, and nervous systems. It is generally accepted that enlargement of a human muscle in training is the result of an increase in the cross-sectional area of the individual muscle cells rather than an increase in the number of muscle cells.

Muscle tissue that is not used will eventually decrease in size. An example of this concept is the loss of muscle size that takes place with a broken arm. When the arm is immobilized by being placed in a cast, the diameter of the limb reduces drastically because of inactivity. This same thing can happen to the total musculature of the human body when an individual becomes sedentary and does not engage in a proper strength program. This loss of muscle tissue can be stopped and an increase in muscle development stimulated by engaging in a strength training program.

Individual muscle cells possess different capacities to contract which are due to inherited characteristics. Muscle cells are classified as either *fast-twitch* cells or *slow-twitch* cells. An individual muscle is composed of both fast-twitch and slow-twitch muscle cells. Fast-twitch cells have the ability to contract very rapidly and thus generate a large amount of force in a short period of time. They expend their energy sources quickly and thus are more easily fatigued.

Slow-twitch cells can exert force for longer periods of time and are used for activities that require submaximum force, such as jogging, walking, and long-distance swimming. Even though genetics determines whether we have muscles composed of a greater percentage of slow-twitch cells or of fast-twitch cells, strength training can affect the ability of both cells to exert force.

It has been determined that proper strength training programs cause the following physiological changes to take place: an increase in the muscle cell filaments used in contraction, an increase in the amount of connective tissue that surrounds the muscle cell and transmits the force of contraction to the bones of the skeletal system, an increase in the chemical properties of the muscle cells that allows for better energy utilization, and an increase in the capillarization of the circulatory system around the muscle cells.

OVERLOAD PRINCIPLE

In any physical fitness program, the *overload principle* is the basic concept that is necessary to bring about improvement in the various systems of the body. As the body is subject to loads greater than those to which the systems are accustomed, the various systems adjust and increase their capacity to perform physical work.

An example of what we are talking about would be the jogger who first runs only one mile and then each week adds another mile to the training program. Because of this overload, certain systems of the body are stimulated and increase their ability to perform the work of jogging. In time the jogger will be able to go ten or more miles on a training run quite easily.

One important fact is that specific body systems require specific overloads, and thus an overload such as that of jogging on the cardiovascular system is different from the overload necessary to bring about strength gains. This is referred to as the *law of specificity*. The minimum resistance that a person can use and still be confident of obtaining strength gains is approximately 60 percent of the maximum force that a muscle group can exert. The following chapters contain all of the information necessary to ensure that the specific overload for strength will be contained in the planning of a strength training program.

BASIC DEFINITIONS

To understand how to organize a strength program, it is necessary to be familiar with the following definitions:

Atrophy: decrease in muscle size

Barbell: a bar with iron plates attached

Bodybuilder: a person who uses weight training to obtain a more muscular physique; a physique athlete

Concentric contraction: a shortening of the muscle against resistance

Dumbbell: a hand weight

Eccentric contraction: a lengthening of the muscle against resistance

Free weights: barbells and dumbbells are known as free weights; free weights differ from strength training machines, which are restricted on how they can be used

Hypertrophy: increase in muscle size

Isokinetic training: the use of a machine that controls the speed of a muscle contraction and attempts to vary the resistance according to the muscle force applied

Isometric contraction: a muscle contraction with little or no movement

Isotonic contraction: muscle contraction with movement

Maximum resistance: maximum weight lifted in one repetition of an exercise

Muscular endurance: the ability to perform repeated muscle movements for a given period of time

Muscular strength: the ability to exert force

Physique: the body structure; organization or development of the physical appearance

Progressive resistance training: increasing the amount of weight lifted as one becomes stronger

Recovery period: the rest interval time between sets

Repetitions: the number of times an exercise is performed

Repetition maximum: the maximum amount of weight lifted for a given number of repetitions. For example, 1

RM would be the maximum weight lifted for one repetition and 6 RM would be the maximum weight lifted for six repetitions

Set: a given number of repetitions

Variable resistance training: the use of a machine that adjusts the resistance through the range of movement of a muscle contraction to accommodate to the change in muscle strength at different joint angles

Weight lifting: competition which requires the participants to use specific lifts

Weight training: a systematic series of resistance exercises to develop strength

STRENGTH PROGRAMS

Many types of training programs can be utilized to develop strength. Any method of training has some advantages and some disadvantages. Regardless of the training method selected, the overload principle must be utilized to obtain strength gains, and the resistance must be progressively increased as the muscles increase in strength.

The classic example is the story told concerning the Greek hero known as Milo of Crotona. Each day he lifted a calf to his shoulders and ran through the stable. As the calf grew and added body weight, this increased weight was the overload needed to bring about the physiological changes in Milo's body systems to make him stronger. This same principle is the cause of increased strength in any training program.

Strength development programs are basically either *isotonic* programs (muscle contractions with movement) or *isometric* programs (muscle contractions with little or no movement).

The most common type of training program is one using isotonic contractions. The major advantage of this system is that it brings about strength gains through a full range of motion. As a muscle goes through a range of motion, it is necessary that it receive adequate resistance at all of the joint angles to stimulate strength increases. For example, if resistance is incurred at only the 90° angle, this is where the muscle will be stronger, not at the other angles, where resistance is not encountered. Isotonic training seems to have a greater effect on muscle hypertrophy, muscle endurance, increased flexibility, and development of connective tissue. Also this type of training allows the individual to observe the work being done, and this can be a source of satisfaction from a psychological standpoint.

From a cosmetic viewpoint, the gains made from an isotonic program are greater than those from an isometric program. Since many people engage in strength programs for body changes related to training, this would be an added plus for isotonic training.

Some advantages ascribed to an isometric training program are that it requires less equipment and usually causes little muscle soreness. It is possible to isolate specific joint angles to strengthen with this mode of training. The author has used specific isometric contractions with the leg muscles to increase the ability of various athletes to jump higher and further. It should be noted that the primary training program for the athletes was isotonic, and the isometric exercises were utilized to supplement this program.

A disadvantage of isometric training is that it causes high systolic and diastolic blood pressures that might be dangerous to the heart and circulatory system.

MACHINES VS. FREE WEIGHTS

In the past few years, as the interest in the development of strength has increased, there has appeared on the market a dazzling array of many different exercise machines. Each advertisement in very convincing language explains why this specific machine is best and why all other machines and training methods will soon be obsolete. Many times the advertisement contains testimonies from prominent athletes or coaches.

With the development of these machines have come new terms in strength training. These are *isokinetic* and *variable resistance*. They are based on the fact that as a muscle goes through a range of motion the ability of the lever system to exert force changes at different angles. Thus the amount of weight that can be lifted is limited by the weakest point in the range of motion. Therefore many manufacturers of equipment have developed machines that theoretically have the ability to adjust the resistance of the machine to the muscle's ability to exert force. The claim is that these machines will bring about a faster and greater increase of strength through the full range of motion.

The other type of training devices are sometimes referred to as *free weights*. Free weights include barbells, dumbbells, and other related equipment. In the early 1900s, Allan Calvert developed the adjustable barbells, with which weighted plates could be added or taken off to change the resistance. In over eighty years, there have been few changes to alter his basic design.

There have been many discussions regarding the merits of the "machines vs. free weights" question, and it may never be answered, in the judgment of some observers. This author takes the stand that it is not an "either or" problem, but a strength trainer should use many different methods in strength training. As long as the basic principles regarding strength development are observed, it is possible to make strength gains and body changes with both machines and free weights. Being consistent in your training in the program you choose is probably more important than the type of program you select. It is recommended that a person experiment with different exercises and various types of training equipment and use them to develop a program that is personalized for that individual's needs.

NUTRITION AND STRENGTH DEVELOPMENT

Nutrition has a significant effect on health. It affects virtually every function of the body. Nutrients from food are necessary for every heartbeat, nerve sensation, and muscle contraction.

Nutrients are chemical substances obtained from food during digestion. About fifty nutrients, including water, are needed daily for optimum health. No single substance will maintain good health. Although specific nutrients are known to have important functions in specific parts of the body, even those nutrients are dependent upon the presence of other nutrients for their best effects. An effort should be made to attain and maintain an adequate, balanced daily intake of all the necessary nutrients throughout life.

For a very simple daily food guide, the United States Department of Agriculture suggests planning the basic diet around four food groups. This guide has the advantages of simplicity and enough freedom of choice to fit individual preferences and different economic levels. Table 2.1 describes the food groups and the servings necessary to provide a well-balanced diet.

Many times a person starting a strength training program becomes concerned about a need for extra protein in the diet. Hoping to increase body size and strength, many individuals have been attracted to high-protein diets and concentrated protein supplements. There is

Table 2.1   Daily Food Guide

Food Group	Examples of Food	Daily Servings
Milk	Milk—cheese, ice cream and other milk-made foods can supply part of the milk	Children: 3 or more glasses Teens: 4 or more glasses Adults: 2 or more glasses
Meat	Meats, fish, poultry, eggs or cheese—dry beans, peas, or nuts as alternates	2 or more servings
Vegetables and Fruits	Include dark green or yellow vegetables; citrus fruit or tomatoes	4 or more servings
Breads and Cereals	Enriched or whole grain Added milk improves nutritional values	4 or more servings

no scientific evidence that supports the belief that people engaging in strength programs require increased amounts of protein. The National Research Council recommends that both men and women consume one gram of protein per kilogram (2.2 lbs.) of body weight. The average American ingests two or three times as much protein as needed. There are some drawbacks to uncontrolled protein intake in the diet. High-protein diets are dehydrating because they demand large amounts of water for urinary excretion of the metabolic by-products. Protein supplements may cause loss of appetite and diarrhea, and excess protein may also be changed to fat, stored in the body and contribute to obesity.

The four food group plan provides abundant protein and is the best nutritional program to follow for a training program.

ANABOLIC STEROIDS

The past years have seen certain individuals take anabolic steroids in the attempt to obtain increased muscle mass and strength. These steroids are artificial male hormones that have anabolic properties, that is, they cause a build-up of complex chemical units, such as muscle protein. There is much contradictory research as to whether the steroids accomplish their intended purpose. Anabolic steroids are banned by every international sports federation, and in some cases athletes have been banned from competition for using these drugs. The position statement that follows from the American College of Sports Medicine details some of the problems associated with their use. A person using anabolic steroids should consult first with a medical doctor and use them only under the doctor's supervision.

Based on a comprehensive survey of the world literature and a careful analysis of the claims made for and against the efficacy of anabolic-androgenic steroids in improving human physical performance, the position of the American College of Sports Medicine is that:

1. The administration of anabolic-androgenic steroids to healthy humans below age 50 in medically approved therapeutic doses often does not of itself bring about any significant improvements in strength, aerobic endurance, lean body mass, or body weight.
2. There is no conclusive scientific evidence that extremely large doses of anabolic-androgenic steroids either aid or hinder athletic performance.
3. The prolonged use of oral anabolic-androgenic steroids (C_{17}-alkylated derivatives of testosterone) has resulted in liver disorders in some persons. Some of these disorders are apparently reversible with the cessation of drug usage, but others are not.
4. The administration of anabolic-androgenic steroids to male humans may result in a decrease in testicular size and function and a decrease in sperm production. Although these effects appear to be reversible when small doses of steroids are used for short periods of time, the reversibility of the effects of large doses over extended periods of time is unclear.
5. Serious and continuing efforts should be made to educate male and female athletes, coaches, physical educators, physicians, trainers, and the general public regarding the inconsistent effects of anabolic-androgenic steroids on improvement of human physical performance and the potential dangers of taking certain forms of these substances, especially in large doses, for prolonged periods.

Variables in the Strength Training Program

A well-designed program to develop strength and reduce the chance of injury must take into consideration the following variables: (1) resistance to utilize; (2) number of repetitions; (3) number of sets; (4) rest interval between sets; (5) frequency of workouts during the week; and (6) safety procedures.

A systematic overloading of a muscle increases the strength and size of the muscle. There are four possible methods that can be used to increase the difficulty of a strength workout. They are:

1. Increase the resistance
2. Increase the repetitions
3. Increase the number of sets
4. Decrease the time of the rest intervals between sets

RESISTANCE

The greatest strength gains seem to be obtained when the resistance is increased and the other variables are held constant. It seems to be that the *minimum* resistance that can be used and still get strength gains is approximately 60 percent of the maximum force or weight lifted for one muscle contraction. The maximum force that can be exerted is referred to as the 1 RM.

It would appear that the fastest way to obtain strength would be to do exercises that would require a single repetition of maximum force. The problem with this type of training is that it may cause injury to the muscle or connective tissue. It may also lead to chronic fatigue of the muscle and retard the progress toward increased strength and muscle development.

REPETITIONS

Resistance exceeding 75 percent of maximum has been found to be very effective in bringing about strength gains in a training program. In comparing the maximum weight lifted in a given exercise, it is found that a 10 RM weightload usually corresponds to approximately 75 percent of that maximum. An example would be a person who can do a single arm curl with 100 pounds, then the 10 RM weightload would be 75 pounds.

A rule of thumb that works well in determining the weightload to use in an exercise is:

Objective is increased muscle strength = decrease the repetitions, increase the resistance.

Objective is increased muscle endurance = increase the repetitions, decrease the resistance.

Thus a football player, who wishes a greater increase in strength, might use 5 RM, and a long distance runner, who needs muscle endurance, might use 15 RM.

Since it becomes difficult to determine exactly how much weight a person should be lifting for each exercise, there is a need for some guidelines to follow. Through the years the author has utilized what is referred to as the "guesstimate" method of determining resistance with great success. This method has been used both with beginning weight training classes and elite athletes. It is basically a process of trial and error.

1. Guess how many pounds you can lift for a specific exercise.
2. Try this weight for the given number of repetitions for one set, i.e., 6 RM, 10 RM, etc.
3. If the exercise is too easy and you can do more than the recommended number of repetitions, increase the resistance for the next set.
4. If the exercise is too hard and you cannot do the recommended number of repetitions, decrease the resistance for the next set.

5. Remember to increase the weight for the next workout whenever you can do more than the recommended number of repetitions on the last set of an exercise.

SETS

The most popular and versatile system of strength development is the set system, in which an individual performs an exercise for a given number of repetitions, rests for an interval of time, and repeats the exercise for a given number of sets. This system can be adapted to any objective in strength development for the beginner, the bodybuilder, the athlete, or the advanced weight lifter.

Most beginning weight trainers make good progress by using a program consisting of three or four sets using 6 to 10 RM in each set.

People who train on the Nautilus machines are recommended to do only one set of 8 to 12 RM. Olympic weightlifters and powerlifters many times train using five to ten sets of 1 to 5 RM each set. Bodybuilders may utilize five to ten sets of 10 to 15 RM in their workouts.

It is recommended that each exercise commence with a warm-up set of a lighter weight. A set of ten repetitions using 50 percent of the maximum weight that can be lifted works very well as a warm-up set. This will help to reduce injury and prepare the muscle system for an additional resistance in the following sets.

REST INTERVAL BETWEEN SETS

The rest interval between sets is an important consideration in the designing of the strength training program. The amount of time taken between sets will be determined by the training objectives of the person. For example, bodybuilders usually take very short rest periods, while weightlifters or athletes training with near to maximum weightloads require relatively extended rest periods between sets.

One of the ways to determine the rest interval is to be aware of the primary energy sources required in the lifting of weights. This energy source, which is composed of the chemicals adenosine triphosphate and phosphocreatine, is known as the phosphagen stores. These phosphagen stores have the ability to provide maximum energy for short periods of time and usually last for no more than ten seconds.

These stores are quickly replenished in the rest interval, and it is estimated that within 30 seconds, approximately 50 percent of the phosphagens are resynthesized and available for another bout of exercise. Table 3.1 contains the amount of rest time and the approximate percentage of phosphagen stores replenished.

Table 3.1   Replenishment of Phosphagen Stores

Rest Time	Approximate Percentage of Phosphagen Stores Replenished
0 seconds	0.00
30 seconds	50.00
60 seconds (1 minute)	75.00
90 seconds	87.50
120 seconds (2 minutes)	93.75
150 seconds	96.88
180 seconds (3 minutes)	98.44
210 seconds	99.22
240 seconds (4 minutes)	99.61
270 seconds	99.80
300 seconds (5 minutes)	99.90

Adapted from Wayne L. Westcott, Ph.D., *Strength Fitness: Physiological Principles and Training Techniques,* Expanded Edition. Copyright © 1983 by Allyn and Bacon, Inc. Used with permission.

As indicated by the table, most of the phosphagen stores are replenished within two minutes. Individuals, such as bodybuilders, who wish to obtain the so-called muscle pump might use one-minute intervals, and those who are lifting near-maximum weight would increase the rest interval to three or more minutes. In most cases, a rest interval of approximately two minutes should be an adequate amount of time.

The recovery is specific to the muscles involved in the exercise, and if a person needs to reduce the time necessary to complete a workout, one could alternate sets of different exercises. For example, do a set using the chest muscles, such as the bench press, and a set utilizing the legs, such as the leg press. Do the exercises until the required number of sets is completed, and then you can move on to two different exercises.

FREQUENCY OF WORKOUTS DURING THE WEEK

When the body systems, such as the muscular system, are overloaded, cells require a certain amount of time to recover and undergo the physiological changes that are involved in training. If the recovery time is too short, the muscle cells are unable to accommodate and rebuild to ensure a higher level of strength. This can lead to chronic fatigue and may even result in a loss of strength. A decrease in performance is the best indicator that a person needs more rest and a decrease in work.

Most strength workouts require a rest day between each workout day for the various muscle groups exercised. A muscle group should be trained on three nonconsecutive days each week, such as Monday, Wednesday, and Friday. In Chapter 7, "Physique Training and Bodybuilding," a type of training will be explained known as the split-body routine, in which a person can work out every day by exercising one part of the body one day then letting it rest while training another body part on the next day.

A person can train any time during the day, and this will usually be determined by the amount of time available and when training facilities can be used.

SAFETY PROCEDURES

An examination of the accidents in various activities reveals that weight training is one of the safest forms of recreation a person can use as a form of participation. Even though this is true, there are some commonsense rules that if followed will reduce the chance of injury.

If a person has been sedentary for a long period and suspects some medical problem, it would be wise to have a good physical examination by a qualified physician.

Fredrick C. Hatfield and March L. Krotee, in their book, *Personalized Weight Training for Fitness and Athletics: From Theory to Practice,* have compiled a list of recommended guidelines that is excellent advice for any weight trainer.

1. Never train alone! Injuries and accidents can often be avoided when someone else is present. It's also more fun to involve others either as a primary or secondary partner. A weight training room should be supervised by trained personnel.

2. Inspect equipment, read instructions and have each piece of equipment demonstrated by a qualified instructor. In short, if you don't know what you're doing, seek professional advice and guidance. Your chances of reaching your training aims and objectives will be greatly enhanced.
3. Use experienced spotters whenever necessary. Heavy squats and bench presses are especially dangerous and under no circumstances should they be attempted without one or two knowledgeable spotters. Other exercises such as good mornings, hyperextensions, and incline or decline presses also require spotting.
4. Keep alert and lift weights or engage in associated physical activity in designated areas only. With multi-use equipment be aware of where you are as well as others around you. Be careful not to walk directly in front of lifters as you may startle them, disturb their concentration, or even inadvertently bump into their equipment.
5. Always check your weights and immediate training environment before each set. Be sure that even loading is followed, collars are tightened and barbell sleeves are free to revolve. Count your weight!
6. Use equipment as it was designed to be employed. Improper use can cause injury, equipment breakdowns, and lost training time.
7. Keep lifting and exercise areas clean, neat and orderly. Place weights in designated areas after using, as misplaced weights are often the cause of injury.
8. When using weight training machines, carefully check all cables, pulleys, selector keys (use appropriate key, not a substitute), nuts, bolts, cam chains, seat adjustments and belts for maximum safety. The equipment should also be kept clean and appropriately lubricated. If equipment jams, do not attempt to free it yourself. Report all problems immediately to the weight training supervisor.
9. Wear proper lifting attire and remember perspiration causes slippery equipment and skin, both dangerous conditions. Don't lift in your stocking feet.
10. Use proper breathing techniques when lifting. If a person takes a deep breath and holds it while straining to lift the weight this can decrease significantly the blood flow to an area of the body. The increased pressure in the chest cavity that can result when holding the breath can hinder the venous blood return to the heart and elevate blood pressure. This is known as the Valsalva effect.

The best system of breathing is to exhale during the lifting movement and inhale during the lowering movement.

11. Don't lift if an injury may be aggravated. Temporarily modify the activity to exclude the injured area or associated muscle group.

12. If you're not feeling well or even up to par, you should temporarily suspend lifting. When recovering from an illness, resume lifting at a level of intensity and weight level well below that achieved before the illness.

13. Attend to weight training through a planned personalized program of progressive resistance training. This will reduce muscle soreness, aching joints and tendons and reduce your chance for injury. Proper technique, supervision in a professionally developed weight training program is mandatory.

14. Be aware of environmental conditions such as room temperature, humidity, altitude, and pollution count and adapt your weight lifting program accordingly.

15. Don't lift immediately after a heavy meal!

16. Excessively hot showers should be avoided immediately after training. In some rare instances, hot showers have been associated with manifestations of myocardial infarction or heart attack.

17. Weight training does not have to be highly competitive in nature to be healthful. In fact, ego in the form of spontaneous and unwarranted 1 RMs like trying to outlift a colleague often leads to a loss of safety focus concerning the physiological boundaries for safe participation.

18. As part of the physiological and psychological preparation for weight training, the warm-up may be considered a safety precaution. Warm-up is a preparation that is conducted at submaximal effort for a duration of approximately five to fifteen minutes immediately before engaging in lifting. Warm-up should be intense enough to increase body temperature and cause perspiration, but should not require a longer duration of submaximal effort. The value of warm-up seems to be quite controversial for participation in various sport specific situations; however, for the individual engaging in regular, vigorous weight training, warm-up is deemed as a vital safety factor.

Body Measurements and Record Keeping

Attempting to reach the goal of strength development can be compared to taking a journey. If you are planning a trip, you need to know where you are starting from and how many miles you have traveled.

By taking your body measurements when you start your program, you will have a means to determine the progress you are making. Record keeping will enable you to evaluate how well the body responds to specific exercises and thus make any changes that might be beneficial to your individual needs. As you compare the increases in resistance used in the various exercises, you also will have a means to determine the strength gains being made by selected body parts.

Taking Measurements

One of the simplest methods to monitor change is to measure the circumference of selected body parts with a tape. When taking the measurements, keep the tape firm, but do not apply enough pressure to make indentations in the skin. By following this procedure, you will have measurements that are reliable and indicate structural changes. All the measurements should be taken in a standing position. In some cases you may wish to take two sets of measurements, one with the body part relaxed and a second with the body part in a flexed position.

Following are some standardized procedures to follow in measuring selected body parts. Figure 4.1 can be used to record the body measurements.

Neck—measure at the smallest circumference when relaxed.
Shoulders—measure the circumference at the greatest width.
Chest—*relaxed,* measure at greatest circumference after
  exhaling.
  flexed, measure at greatest circumference after inhaling.

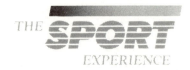

Use the Body Measurement Chart to record your body measurements. After you have engaged in your strength training program for three or more months, take the measurements again to determine how your body is changing.

Upper Arm—*relaxed*, measure at largest circumference with arm hanging.

flexed, measure at largest circumference with elbow at a 90° angle.

Forearm—*relaxed*, measure largest circumference with arm hanging.

flexed, measure largest circumference while flexing muscles by bending the elbow and the wrist.

Waist—measure at smallest circumference after exhaling.

Hips—measure at largest circumference.

Thigh—*relaxed*, measure the largest circumference.

flexed, measure the largest circumference while straightening the leg and contracting the thigh muscles.

Calf—*relaxed*, measure the largest circumference.

flexed, measure the largest circumference while contracting the muscles of the lower leg by raising the heel.

Keeping a Record

Now that you have your body measurements, you have a means to plot your progress as you engage in your training program. Compiling a strength training record can also be a tremendous aid in your program. This record enables you to know the exercise you are using and the exact poundage to lift for that exercise. By comparing the various exercise days, you can easily determine how much improvement you have made at any given time. Figure 4.2 is an example of a strength training record. Additional body measurement charts and strength training records can be found in Appendices B and C.

Figure 4.1 Body Measurement Chart

Name _____ Age _____

Date											
Body Weight											
Neck											
Shoulders											
Chest	Relaxed										
	Flexed										
Upper Arm Relaxed	Right										
	Left										
Flexed	Right										
	Left										
Forearm Relaxed	Right										
	Left										
Flexed	Right										
	Left										
Waist											
Hips											
Thigh Relaxed	Right										
	Left										
Flexed	Right										
	Left										
Calf Relaxed	Right										
	Left										
Flexed	Right										
	Left										
Other Body Parts											

Body Measurements and Record Keeping

Figure 4.2 Strength Training Record

Name _____   Age _____

Date					
Exercise	Wt Reps	Wt Reps	Wt Reps	Wt Reps	Wt Reps

STRENGTH TRAINING

Wt Reps	Wt Reps	Wt Reps	Wt Reps	Wt Reps	Wt Reps

Body Measurements and Record Keeping

Planning the Strength Training Program

In planning a strength training program to ensure overall body strength and development, there are six major body parts that should be included in the program. These are (1) neck, (2) arms (biceps, triceps, and shoulders), (3) chest, (4) back, (5) midsection, and (6) legs.

When designing the program, the individual must be aware of the equipment available and the amount of training time that he or she has. The desired outcomes to be achieved by the program should also be known.

At the end of this chapter, in the photo section, are descriptions of the various exercises that can be employed. There are pictures showing the exercise, and, in addition, there is an explanation concerning the starting position of the exercise, the action to be followed, and any precautions to be aware of while doing the exercise.

Table 5.1 lists the six major body parts and the exercises that will strengthen the muscles in these body parts. By using this table you can select exercises to develop any part of the body. Please note that although an exercise is listed under one area, as the bench press is under the chest area, it will also involve other parts of the body such as the arms.

Table 5.1 follows this page. Following Table 5.1 is an example of a beginning strength training program.

Table 5.1   Weight Training Exercises

Body Part	Exercise	Page Located
1. Neck	Neck strap	30
	Partner resistance	31
	Wrestler's bridge	32
2. Arms and Shoulders		
Biceps	Arm curl	33
	Reverse curl	34
	Preacher-board curl	35
	Dumbbell curl	36
	Incline dumbbell curl	37
	Dumbbell concentration curl	38
	Supine curl	39
Triceps	Standing overhead press	40
	Seated overhead press	41
	Behind-neck press	42
	Seated behind-neck press	43
	Standing dumbbell press	44
	Seated dumbbell press	45
	Lying barbell triceps extension	46
	Standing barbell triceps extension	47
	Lying dumbbell triceps extension	48
	Seated dumbbell triceps extension	49
	Dumbbell kickback	50
	Triceps pressdown	51
Wrists	Wrist curl	52
	Reverse wrist curl	53
	Dumbbell wrist curl	54
	Reverse dumbbell wrist curl	55
	Wrist roller	56
Shoulders	Upright rowing	57
	Side lateral raises	58
	Dips	59
	Seated dips	60
3. Chest	Barbell bench press	61
	Dumbbell bench press	62
	Barbell incline bench press	63
	Dumbbell incline bench press	64
	Bench flys	65
	Bent-arm flys	66
	Decline press	67
	Bent-arm pullover	68

By using the following plan you can design a program using one exercise per body part. If you wish, you can add more exercises for selected body parts.

Body Part	Exercise	Sets	Repetitions	Rest Interval
Chest	Bench Press	3	10 RM	2 minutes
Midsection	Curl-ups	3	30 RM	2 minutes
Triceps	Triceps pressdown	3	10 Rm	2 minutes
Legs	Leg press	3	10 RM	2 minutes
Shoulders	Dips	3	10 RM	2 minutes
Neck	Partner resistance	3	10 RM	2 minutes
Biceps	Arm curl	3	10 RM	2 minutes
Legs	Leg curl	3	10 RM	2 minutes
Back	Lat-pulldown	3	10 RM	2 minutes

Strength Training Worksheet

Name _____

Body Part	Exercise	Sets	Reps	Resistance
Chest				
Midsection				
Triceps				
Legs				
Shoulders				
Neck				
Biceps				
Back				

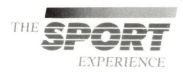

THE SPORT EXPERIENCE

Write an individualized strength training program for yourself using the Strength Training Worksheet.

Planning the Strength Training Program

NECK EXERCISES

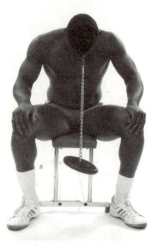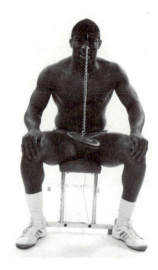

Neck Strap

Starting Position: Place the strap on the head, and take a seated position on the bench.

Action:
A. Muscles on the back of the neck: Bend over slightly at the waist, and move the head forward and backward. Allow the weight to hang between the legs.
B. Muscle on the front of the neck: Bend slightly backward, and move the head forward and backward. Allow the weight to hang behind the back.
C. Muscles on the side of the neck: Lean slightly to the right, and move the head from side to side. Allow the weight to hang to the right side of the body. When you have completed the desired number of repetitions, move the weight to the left side of the body and repeat the exercise.

Precautions: Since the neck muscles are usually quite weak, start with higher repetitions and light weights. Do not jerk the weight or use unnecessary body motion in the movement.

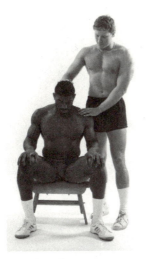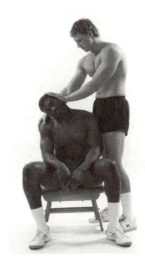

Partner Resistance

Starting Position: Take a seated position on the bench.

Action: To provide resistance the partner pushes against the head as the neck muscles contract in the various positions: forward, backward, and sideways.

Precautions: Be sure to exercise all the neck muscles. Do not jerk the head in the movement.

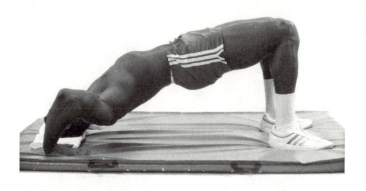

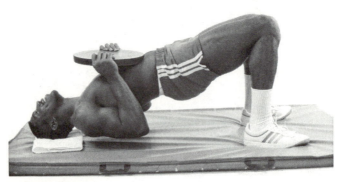

Wrestler's Bridge

Starting Position: Lie flat on your back with your head resting on a pad. Pull the feet in close to the buttocks until the weight of the body is supported by the head and the feet.

Action: Rotate the body on the head using a forward and backward and side-to-side motion.

Precautions: Do not use a jerky movement.

NOTE: To increase the resistance, weights can be placed on the chest or a partner can push against the chest while the exercise is done.

BICEPS EXERCISES

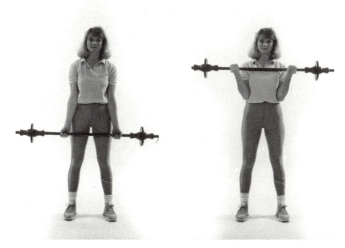

Arm Curl

Starting Position: Grasp the bar about the width of the shoulders using a palms-up grip. The arms are extended, and the bar rests against
the thighs.

Action: Curl the bar up to the shoulder area. Touch, and then return
to the starting position.

Precautions: The elbows should be kept close to the sides of the body.
Keep the body erect with the head up. Avoid any unnecessary body
movement.

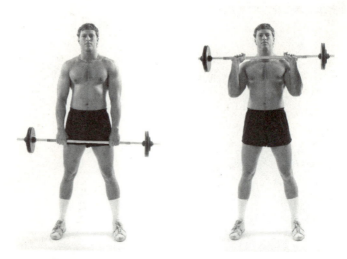

Reverse Curl

Starting Position: Grasp the bar about the width of the shoulders using a palms-down grip. The arms are extended, and the bar rests against the thighs.

Action: Curl the bar up to the shoulder area. Touch, and then return to the starting position.

Precautions: The elbows should be kept close to the sides of the body. Keep the body erect with the head up. Avoid any unnecessary body movement.

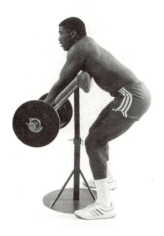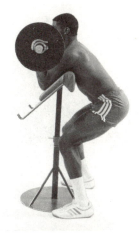

Preacher-Board Curl

Starting Position: Adjust the stand to a height where you can place your arms over the angled padding with the back of the arms resting on the pad. Grasp the bar about the width of the shoulders using a palms-up grip.

Action: Curl the bar up to the shoulder area. Touch, and then return to the starting position.

Precautions: Do not jerk the weight and avoid any unnecessary body movement.

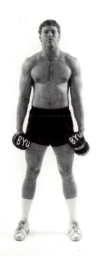 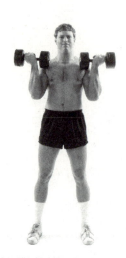

Dumbbell Curl

Starting Position: Stand erect with the feet about shoulder width. Grasp the dumbbells with a palms-up grip with the arms fully extended.

Action: Curl the dumbbells until they reach the top of the shoulders. Touch and return to the starting position.

Precautions: Keep the elbows close to the body. Do not jerk or use any unnecessary motion in the movement.

NOTE: This exercise can be performed in a seated position and also done by alternating one arm then the other in the curling movement.

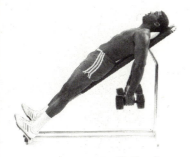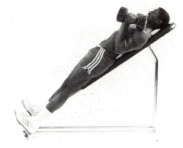

Incline Dumbbell Curl

Starting Position: Lie on an incline board while grasping the dumb-bells in a palms-up grip. The arms are extended with the head and back against the board.

Action: Curl the dumbbells until they reach the shoulders. Touch, and return to the starting position.

Precautions: Do not arch the back or use the legs in the movement. Do not jerk the weight to start the motion.

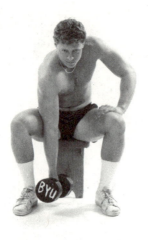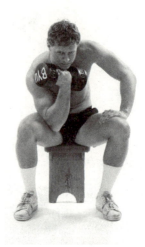

Dumbbell Concentration Curl

Starting Position: Take a seated position on the bench. Grasp the dumbbell in a palms-up grip, and place the elbow on the inside of the right thigh to stabilize the upper arm. The arm is fully extended. The left hand is placed on the left thigh for support.

Action: Curl the dumbbell to the shoulder. Touch, and return to the starting position. After completing the desired number of repetitions, change the dumbbell to the left hand to complete the exercise for both arms.

Precautions: Keep the upper torso and legs stationary during the exercise. Do not jerk the dumbbell, and avoid any unnecessary motion during the movement.

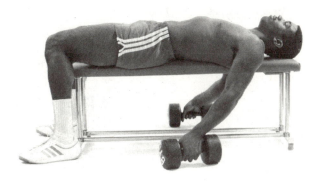

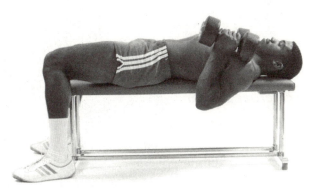

Supine Curl

Starting Position: Lie on the bench with the feet flat on the floor. Grasp the dumbbells with a palms-up grip. The arms are extended from the sides of the body toward the floor.

Action: Curl the dumbbells to the shoulders. Touch, and return to the starting position.

Precautions: Do not arch the back or use any unnecessary motion during the movement.

TRICEPS EXERCISES

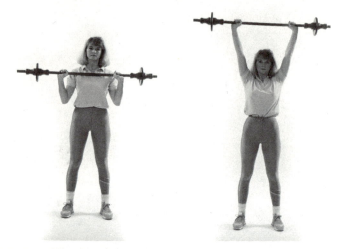

Standing Overhead Press

Starting Position: Stand erect with the feet shoulder width apart. The head is up with the eyes facing straight ahead. The bar rests at the midline of the chest; a palms-up grip is used.

Action: Push the bar overhead until the arms are fully extended. Lower the bar to the starting position.

Precautions: Keep the head up and the back straight. Do not bend the knees to assist the upper-body muscles in the movement.

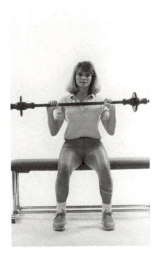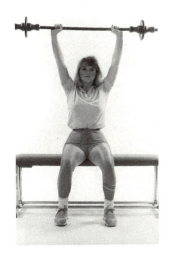

Seated Overhead Press

Starting Position: Take a seat on the bench with the feet flat on the floor. Use a palms-up grip with the bar placed at the midline of the chest. The head is up and the back sraight.

Action: Push the bar overhead until the arms are fully extended. Return to the starting position.

Precautions: Do not jerk the weight or use any unnecessary body motion in the movement.

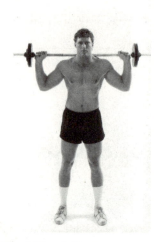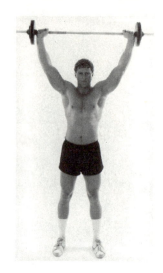

Behind-Neck Press

Starting Position: Stand erect with the feet shoulder width apart. The head is up with the eyes facing straight ahead. The bar is behind the neck and across the shoulders and held with an overhand grip.

Action: Push the bar overhead until the arms are fully extended. Lower the bar to the starting position.

Precautions: Keep the body erect during the exercise. Do not bend the knees to assist the upper-body muscles in the movement.

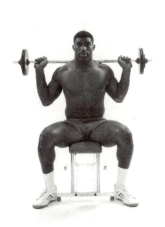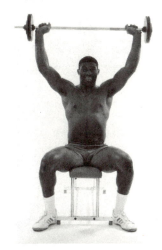

Seated Behind-Neck Press

Starting Position: Take a seat on the bench with the feet flat on the floor. The head is up with the eyes facing straight ahead. The bar is behind the neck and across the shoulders and held with an overhand grip.

Action: Push the bar overhead until the arms are fully extended. Lower the bar to the starting position.

Precautions: Do not jerk the weight or use any unnecessary body motion during the movement.

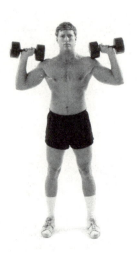 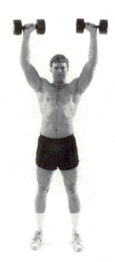

Standing Dumbbell Press

Starting Position: Stand erect with the feet shoulder width apart. Grasp the dumbbells, and bring them to the shoulders with the palms facing forward.

Action: Push the dumbbell overhead until the arms are fully extended. Lower the dumbbells to the starting position.

Precautions: Do not jerk the dumbbells or bend the knees to assist in the movement. Keep the body erect during the motion.

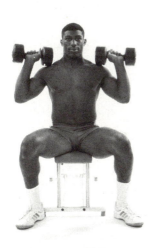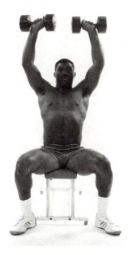

Seated Dumbbell Press

Starting Position: Take a seat on the bench with the feet flat on the floor. Grasp the dumbbells, and bring them to the shoulders with the palms facing forward.

Action: Push the dumbbells overhead until the arms are fully extended. Lower the dumbbells to the starting position.

Precautions: Do not jerk the dumbbells or use any unnecessary body motion in the movement.

NOTE: This exercise can also be performed by alternating one arm then the other in the pressing movement.

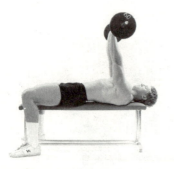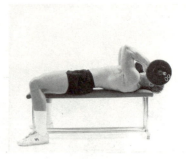

Lying Barbell Triceps Extension

Starting Position: Lie flat on the bench with the feet flat on the floor. Grasp the bar with a narrow overhand grip so that the hands are about six inches or less apart. The arms are fully extended above the chest.

Action: Keep the upper arms extended, and lower the bar until it touches the forehead. Return to the starting position.

Precautions: Do not arch the body or allow the elbows to flare out to the sides during the movement.

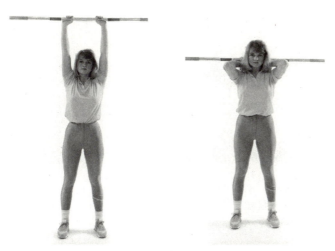

Standing Barbell Triceps Extension

Starting Position: Stand erect with the feet shoulder width apart. Grasp the bar with a narrow overhand grip so that the hands are about six inches or less apart. The arms are fully extended above the head.

Action: Keep the upper arms stationary, and lower the bar until it touches the back of the neck. Return to the starting position.

Precautions: Do not jerk the weight or bend the knees to assist in the lift. Do not allow the elbows to flare out to the sides during the movement.

NOTE: This exercise can also be performed in a seated position.

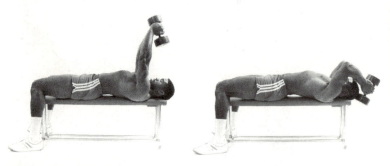

Lying Dumbbell Triceps Extension

Starting Position: Lie flat on the bench with the feet flat on the floor. Grasp the dumbbell in both hands with the fingers interlaced. The arms are fully extended above the chest.

Action: Keep the upper arms extended, and lower the dumbbell until it touches the back of the head. Return to the starting position.

Precautions: Do not arch the body or allow the elbows to flare out to the sides during the movement.

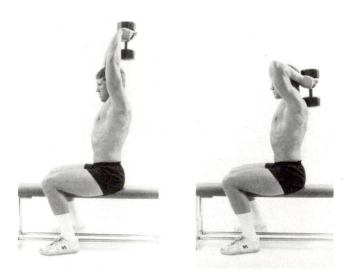

Seated Dumbbell Triceps Extension

Starting Position: Take a seat on the bench with the feet flat on the floor. Grasp the dumbbell in both hands with the fingers interlaced. The arms are fully extended above the head.

Action: Keep the upper arms extended, and lower the dumbbell until it touches the back of the neck. Return to the starting position.

Precautions: Do not jerk the dumbbell or allow the elbows to flare out to the sides during the movement.

NOTE: Dumbbell triceps extensions can also be done in a standing position, or the exercise can be performed using a dumbbell held in one hand at a time.

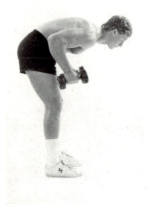
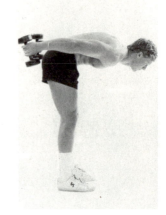

Dumbbell Kickback

Starting Position: Bend over at the waist until the upper torso is parallel to the floor. The feet are shoulder width apart. Grasp the dumbbells in both hands so that the palms are facing each other. The upper arms are parallel to the floor, and the forearms are bent at a 45° angle to the upper arms.

Action: Straighten both arms to the back until the elbows lock. Return to the starting position.

Precautions: Keep the body stationary, and do not jerk the dumbbells in the movement.

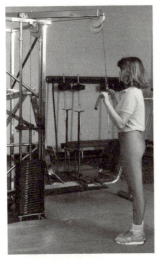 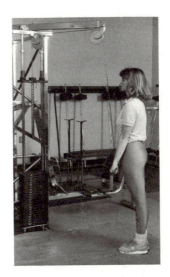

Triceps Pressdown

Starting Position: Stand erect with the feet shoulder width apart. Grasp the bar of the machine with a palms-down grip with the hands about six inches apart. The bar is chest height.

Action: Keep the upper arms stationary, and push the bar to the thighs by extending the forearms. Touch, and return to the starting position.

Precautions: Lean slightly in toward the bar while doing the exercise. Do not move the body to assist the triceps in extending the bar. Keep the elbows close to the body.

WRIST EXERCISES

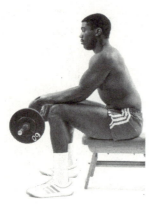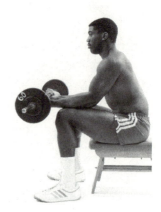

Wrist Curl

Starting Position: Take a seat on the bench with the feet flat on the floor. Grasp the bar with a palms-up grip, and support the arms on the thighs with the wrists extended beyond the knees. The wrists are relaxed so the bar is as low to the floor as possible.

Action: Curl the weight upward as high as possible without moving the forearms. Return to the starting position.

Precautions: Do not jerk the weight, and make sure nothing but the wrists moves during the exercise.

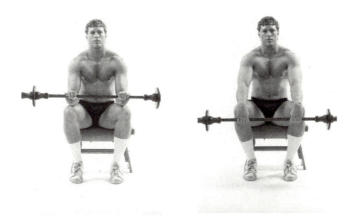

Reverse Wrist Curl

Starting Position: Take a seat on the bench with the feet flat on the floor. Grasp the bar with a palms-down grip, and support the arms on the thighs with the wrists extended beyond the knees. The wrists are relaxed so the bar is as low to the floor as possible.

Action: Curl the weight upward as high as possible without moving the forearms. Return to the starting position.

Precautions: Do not jerk the weight, and make sure nothing but the wrists moves during the exercise.

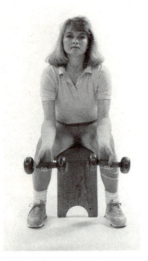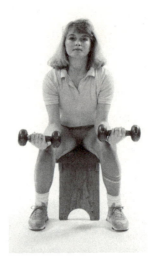

Dumbbell Wrist Curl

Starting Position: Take a seat on the bench with the feet flat on the floor. Grasp the dumbbell in each hand with a palms-up grip, and support the arms on the thighs with the wrists extended beyond the knees. The wrists are relaxed so the dumbbells are as low to the floor as possible.

Action: Curl the dumbbells upward as high as possible without moving the forearms. Return to the starting position.

Precautions: Do not jerk the weight, and make sure nothing but the wrists moves during the exercise.

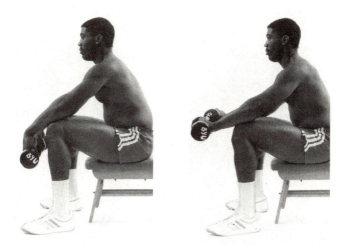

Reverse Dumbbell Wrist Curl

Starting Position: Take a seat on the bench with the feet flat on the floor. Grasp the dumbbell in each hand with a palms-down grip, and support the arms on the thighs with the wrists extended beyond the knees. The wrists are relaxed so the dumbbells are as low to the floor as possible.

Action: Curl the dumbbells upward as high as possible without moving the forearms. Return to the starting position.
.

Precautions: Do not jerk the weight, and make sure nothing but the wrists moves during the exercise.

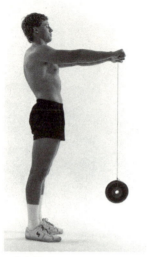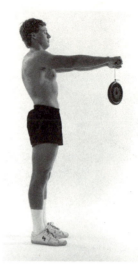

Wrist Roller

Starting Position: Stand erect with the feet about shoulder width apart. Grasp the bar with a palms-down grip with the hands approximately eight inches apart. The wrist roller consists of a weight attached to a bar by a three-foot length of rope. The arms are extended forward and parallel to the floor.

Action: Rotate the hands about the bar until all of the rope is wrapped around the bar. Return to the starting position.

Precautions: Do not move the body to assist in the movement, and do not allow the weight to drop on the extention because this could burn the hands.

NOTE: A clockwise rotation develops the wrist flexors, and a counter-clockwise rotation develops the wrist extensors.

SHOULDER EXERCISES

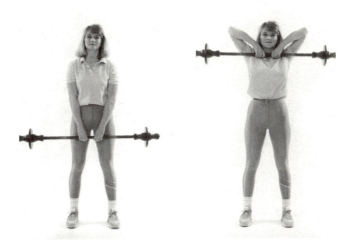

Upright Rowing

Starting Position: Stand erect with the feet about shoulder width apart. Grasp the bar with a palms-down grip with the hands about two inches apart. The arms are extended so the bar rests against the thighs.

Action: Keep the head up and the chest high. Raise the bar until it touches the chin. Return to the starting position.

Precautions: Do not move the body to assist in the exercise. Keep the bar close to the body with the elbows higher than the hands, and don't jerk to start the movement.

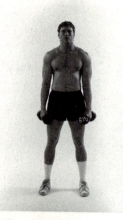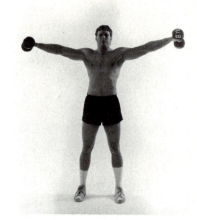

Side Lateral Raise

Starting Position: Stand erect with the feet about shoulder width apart. Grasp a dumbbell in each hand using an overhand grip. The arms are extended downward in front of the body.

Action: Raise the dumbbells upward to the sides of the body until the elbows lock and the arms are approximately parallel to the floor. Return to the starting position.

Precautions: Keep the body stationary, and do not jerk the dumbbells in the movement.

NOTE: You can vary the hand grip. As you change the palms from downward to upward, resistance is moved from the medial deltoid to the anterior deltoid.

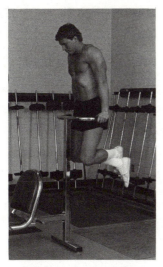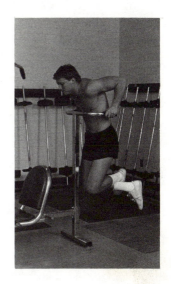

Dips

Starting Position: The body is supported in a suspended position between the parallel bars with the arms fully extended.

Action: Dip downward as far as possible. Return to the starting position.

Precautions: Avoid unnecessary body swing in the movement. Add weights to the body to increase the resistance, if needed.

NOTE: If it is not possible to do the dip as described, the resistance can be decreased as shown in the following pictures.

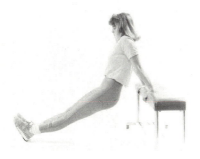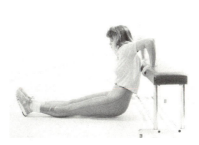

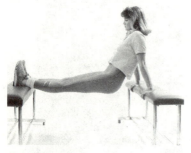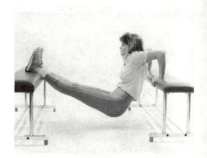

Seated Dips

Starting Position: The body is supported on two benches by placing the feet on one bench and the hands on the other. The arms are fully extended, and the back is straight.

Action: Bend the arms, and allow the body to lower as far as possible. Return to the starting position.

Precautions: Avoid unnecessary body movement in performing the exercise. Weights can be placed on the upper thighs to increase the resistance, if needed.

CHEST EXERCISES

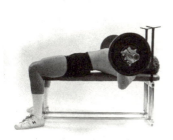 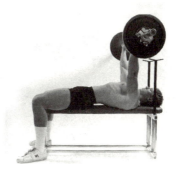

Barbell Bench Press

Starting Position: Lie flat on the bench with the knees bent and feet flat on the floor. Use a palms-up grip, approximately the width of the shoulders. Hold the bar in a chest-rest position.

Action: Press the bar directly upward until elbows lock, and then return to the starting position.

Precautions: Do not arch the back or raise the buttocks during movement. Do not bounce the weight off chest.

NOTE: This exercise can be done using a narrow grip to increase resistance to the triceps.

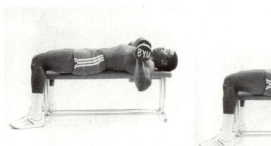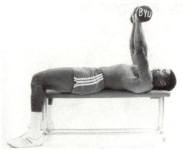

Dumbbell Bench Press

Starting Position: Lie flat on the bench with the knees bent and feet flat on the floor. Grasp the dumbbells with a palms-up grip. Hold the dumbbells in a chest-rest position.

Action: Press the dumbbells directly upwards until elbows lock, and return to the starting position.

Precautions: Do not arch the back or raise the buttocks during movement. Keep the elbows away from the body and pointed outward.

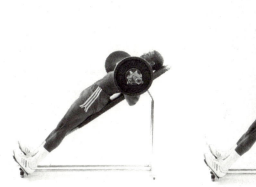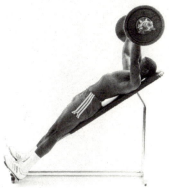

Barbell Incline Bench Press

Starting Position: Lie flat on inclined bench with legs straight and feet flat against supports. Use a palms-up grip, approximately the width of the shoulders. Hold the bar in a chest-rest position.

Action: Press the bar upward until elbows lock, and then return to the starting position.

Precautions: Do not arch the back or raise the buttocks during movement. Do not bounce weight off the chest.

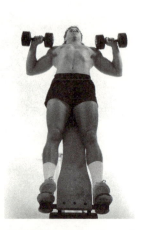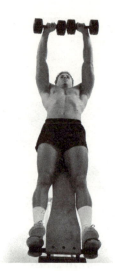

Dumbbell Incline Bench Press

Starting Position: Lie flat on inclined bench with legs straight and feet flat against supports. Grasp the dumbbells with a palms-up grip, and hold them in a chest-rest position.

Action: Press the dumbbells upward until the elbows lock, and then return to the starting position.

Precautions: Do not arch the back or raise the buttocks during the movement. Keep the elbows away from the body and pointed outward.

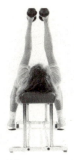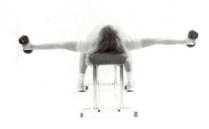

Bench Flys

Starting Position: Lie flat on bench. Hold dumbbell in each hand, straight up over the chest with the palms inward.

Action: Lower the dumbbells with the arms straight until the arms are parallel to the floor, and then return to the starting position.

Precautions: Do not arch the back or raise the buttocks. Lower and raise the dumbbells slowly.

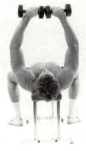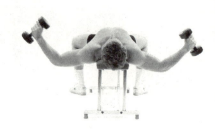

Bent-Arm Flys

Starting Position: Lie flat on bench. Hold a dumbbell in each hand with the arms extended over the chest in a semi-flexed position.

Action: Lower the dumbbells with the arms semi-flexed, as far as they can go toward the floor. Return to starting position.

Precautions: Keep the arms semi-flexed. Do not arch the back or raise the buttocks. Lower and raise the dumbbells slowly.

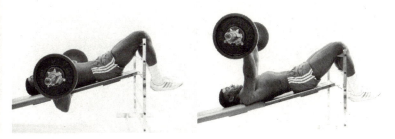

Decline Press

Starting Position: Lie back on a 30° decline bench with the head at the lower end and the knees hooked over the top of bench. Use a palms-up grip approximately the width of the shoulder. Hold the bar in a chest-rest position.

Action: Press the bar upward at approximately 60° until elbows lock, and then return to starting position.

Precautions: Do not arch the back or raise the buttocks during movement. Do not bounce weight off chest.

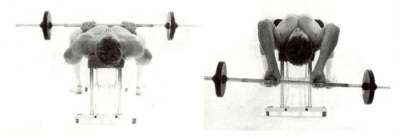

Bent-Arm Pullover

Starting Position: Lie flat on bench with knees bent and feet flat on the floor. Allow head to hang over the end of the bench. Use a palms-up grip with the hands approximately 12 inches apart. Hold the bar in a chest-rest position.

Action: Lower the bar back overhead as far as possible with the elbows bent. Pull the weight back to the starting position.

Precautions: Keep elbows close to the head and pointing toward the ceiling during the exercise. Avoid unnecessary arching of back. Do not jerk or make unnecessary body movements. Keep the bar close to face during the exercise movement.

BACK EXERCISES

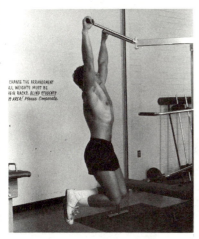 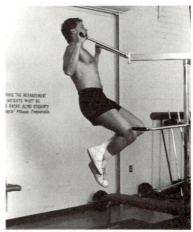

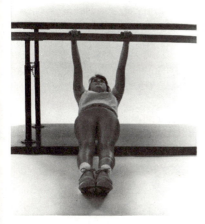 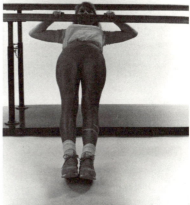

Pull-Up

Starting Position: Use a palms-down grip, approximately the width of the shoulders, with arms extended to support body suspended from the bar.

Action: Pull body upward to the bar until the chin is above the bar, and then return to starting position.

Precautions: Straighten out arms on each repetition. Avoid unnecessary body swing and movement. Add weights to body to increase the resistance, if needed.

NOTE: If you cannot do the pull-up as described, it is possible to decrease the resistance as shown in the second set of pictures.

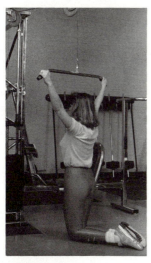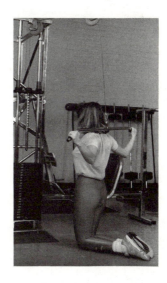

Lat-Pulldown

Starting Position: Start in a kneeling or seated position. Grasp bar in a wide palms-down grip with arms fully extended.

Action: Pull the bar down until it touches the base of the neck, and then return to the starting position.

Precautions: Keep the upper body straight. Do not jerk or raise body to assist in the movement.

NOTE: The same exercise can be done but with the bar pulled downward in front of the chest.

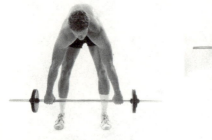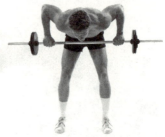

Bent-Over Rowing

Starting Position: Start in a bent-over position with the upper torso parallel to the floor. The feet are shoulder width apart with the knees slightly bent. Grasp the bar with an overhand grip with the arms fully extended.

Action: Pull the bar upward until it touches the rib cage, and then return to the starting position.

Precautions: Keep the spine in an arched position to take pressure off the lower back. Do not jerk the weight or raise the body to assist in the movement.

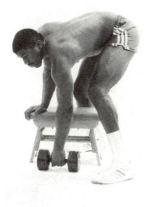 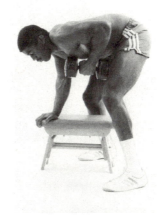

Dumbbell Bent-Over Rowing

Starting Position: Start in a bent-over position with the upper torso parallel to the floor. The feet are shoulder width apart with the knees slightly bent. Grasp the dumbbell with the arm fully extended, the opposite arm supporting the body by contacting a bench for stability.

Action: Pull the dumbbell upward until it touches the torso, and then return to the starting position.

Precautions: Keep the elbow close the body while doing the exercise. Do not jerk the weight or raise the body to assist in the movement.

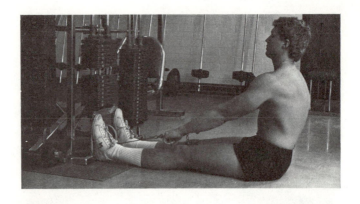

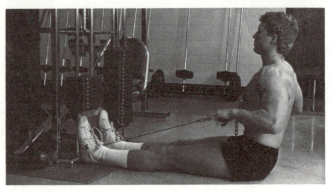

Seated Rowing

Starting Position: Take a seated position with the legs fully extended and braced against the machine. Grasp the bar with a palms-down grip and the arms extended.

Action: Pull the bar toward the body until it touches the lower chest, and then return to the starting position.

Precautions: Keep the back straight during the exercise. Do not jerk to assist in the movement.

NOTE: This exercise can be done with a palms-up grip, which will utilize the biceps of the arm to a greater amount.

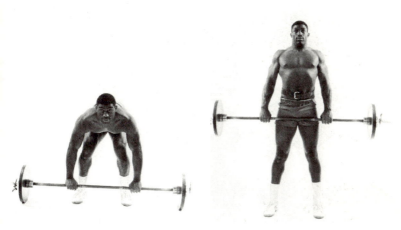

Dead Lift

Starting Position: Stand next to the bar with the front of legs touching the bar and the feet shoulder width apart. Bend down and grasp the bar with the palms facing toward the legs and the hands about shoulder width apart. Bend the legs with the hips lowered and head up. Arch the back to take stress off the lower back.

Action: Pull the bar up along the legs until the body is upright and the bar is on the front of the thighs.

Precautions: Keep the bar close to the legs to reduce back strain. Always keep the head up and lift with the legs.

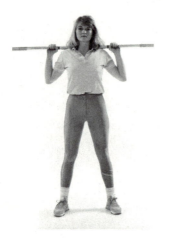
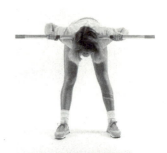

Good Morning

Starting Position: Stand with the bar behind the neck and resting on the shoulders. The feet are shoulder width apart with the legs straight.

Action: Bend forward at the waist until the upper torso is parallel with the floor, and then return to the starting position.

Precautions: Since this exercise puts stress on the lower back muscles, it is important to start with light resistance at first. Keep the head up at all times, and do not jerk to assist in the movement.

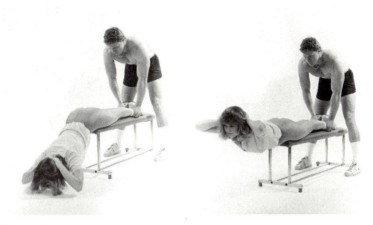

Back Raise

Starting Position: Take a prone position on a bench with the lower part of the body on the bench and the upper torso bent forward over the bench. The hands are interlocked behind the neck. It may be necessary to have a partner support the lower body by pushing down on the legs.

Action: Raise the upper torso upward until the body is parallel to the floor, and then return to the starting position.

Precautions: Do not hyperextend the back by going above parallel. Do not jerk or use any unnecessary motion to assist in the movement.

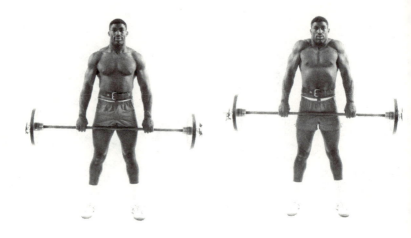

Shrugs

Starting Position: Stand upright and grasp the bar with a palms-down grip with the arms fully extended.

Action: Elevate the shoulder girdle as high as possible, and then return to the starting position.

Precautions: Keep the body straight, and do not bend the arms when raising the weight.

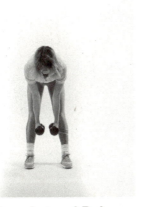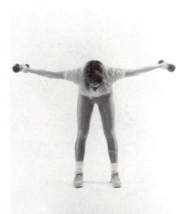

Bent-Over Lateral Raise

Starting Position: Start in a bent-over position with the upper torso parallel to the floor. The feet are shoulder width apart with the knees slightly bent. Grasp the dumbbells in each hand with the arms fully extended.

Action: Raise the dumbbells lateral from the body until the arms are parallel to the floor, and then return to the starting position.

Precautions: Keep the head up, and do not jerk the weight or raise the body to assist in the movement.

MIDSECTION EXERCISES

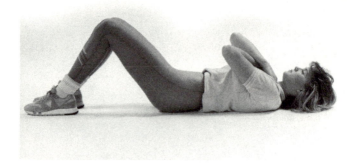

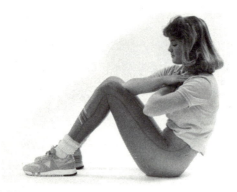

Curl-Up

Starting Position: Lie flat on the floor, with legs bent at the knees and the feet flat on the floor. The hands are folded over the chest.

Action: Curl up to approximately a 30° angle. Rotate the right side of body toward left knee, and return to starting position. On the next repetition rotate body toward right knee.

Precautions: Do not stabilize the feet unless absolutely necessary. Do not arch the back during the exercise, and keep the arms flat against the chest. Be sure to start by bending the head forward and progressively curl-up to the 30° angle. Curl back to the starting position by touching lower back, upper back, and finally the head. A good check is to have someone place a hand under the lower back; the body should press down on the hand until the lower back is curled forward.

NOTE: If the curl-up cannot be done as described, it is possible to decrease the resistance by placing the hands alongside the hips instead of over the chest. To increase the resistance, weights can be held on the chest while doing the exercise. Another method to increase the resistance is to use an incline board and to raise the board to provide a greater amount of resistance.

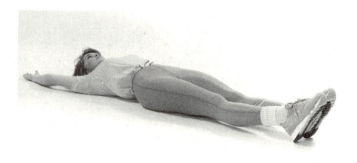

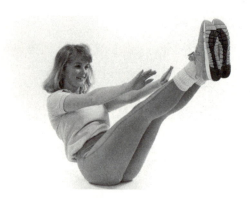

V-Sit

Starting Position: Lie flat on the floor with the legs straight and the arms fully extended above the head.

Action: Raise the legs and arms at the same time, and touch the hands and feet together above the body. Hold this position for one second and return to the starting position.

Precautions: Keep the arms and legs straight while doing the exercise. Do not jerk or make any unnecessary motion to assist in the movement.

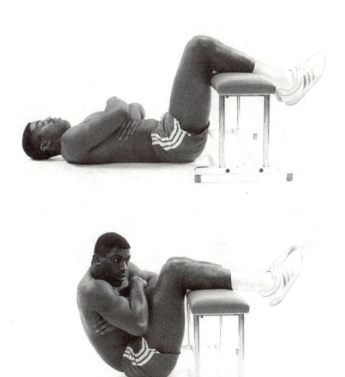

Roman Chair Curl-Up

Starting Position: Lie flat on the floor with knees bent over a bench. The hands are folded over the chest. To increase resistance, weights can be held on the chest.

Action: Curl up and rotate the body until right side of body touches left knee and return to start position. On next repetition rotate body to the right knee.

Precautions: Do not arch back during the curl-up. Do not jerk the body during the movement.

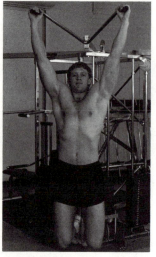 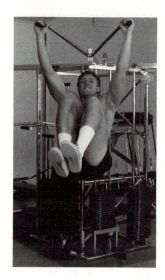

Hanging Knee-Up

Starting Position: Grasp the bar and allow the body to be completely extended.

Action: Raise the legs, knees bent, until the knees touch the chest, and return to the starting position.

Precautions: Raise the legs slowly without jerking to assist in the movement.

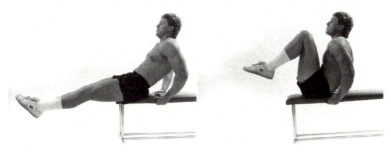

Sitting Knee-Up

Starting Position: Sit on the end of the bench with the legs extended away from the bench. Lean the upper torso back and grasp the bench with the hands.

Action: Slowly bend your knees and raise them to the chest. Touch the knees against the chest, and return to the starting position.

Precautions: Hold the feet and knees together during the exercise. Do not jerk the body during the movement.

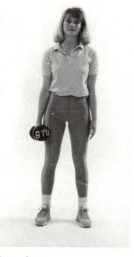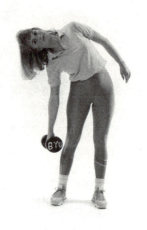

Side Bend

Starting Position: Stand upright with a dumbbell held in one hand and the arms completely extended.

Action: Bend sideways as far as possible toward the side with the dumbbell and return to the starting position. When the desired number of repetitions have been completed, change the dumbbell to the other hand and repeat the exercise to the other side.

Precautions: Do not jerk the weight or use any unnecessary motion in the movement.

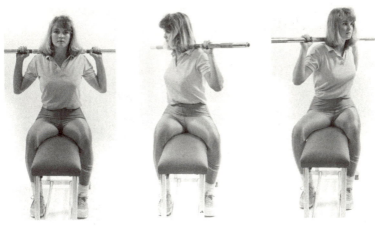

Twists

Starting Position: Take a straddle seated position on a bench with the back straight and the head looking forward. Place the bar behind the neck and across the shoulders.

Action: Keep the pelvic region locked and twist the upper torso as far as possible to the right. Return to the starting position, and then twist to the left and return to the starting position.

Precautions: Squeeze with the knees against the bench to keep the hips from rotating. Do not jerk the body during the movement.

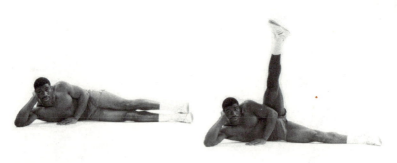

Leg Splits

Starting Position: Lie flat on the right side of the body with the right hand and arm under the head. Use the left arm to support the body in the proper position during the exercise.

Action: Raise the left leg as high as possible and return to the starting position. When the desired number of repetitions have been completed on the right side, change to the left side and repeat the exercise.

Precautions: Keep the leg straight at all times, and do not jerk the body in the movement.

NOTE: To increase the resistance, weights can be added to the feet and ankles.

LEG EXERCISES

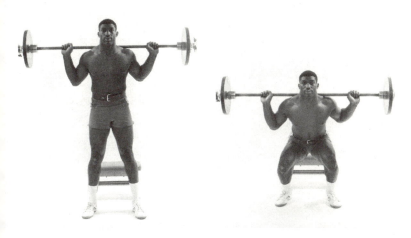

Squat

Starting Position: Stand erect with the feet about shoulder width apart. Place the bar behind the neck and across the shoulders. Keep the head up and the back straight.

Action: Lower the body until the thighs are parallel with the floor. Return to the starting position.

Precautions: Have partners assist as spotters during the exercise. Keep back straight and chest high throughout the movement. Rounding the back can place stress on spine and cause injury. Do not bounce at the bottom of the squat. As a safety device, place a bench behind the lifter that will allow one to sit down if balance is lost.

NOTE: This exercise can be performed at any selected joint angle depending on the needs of the person training.

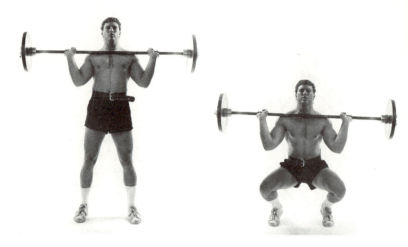

Front Squat

Starting Position: Stand erect with the feet about shoulder width apart. Hold the bar in front of the neck and across the shoulders. Support the bar by wrapping the hands around the middle of the bar with an overhand grip. Keep the head up and the back straight.

Action: Lower the body until the thighs are parallel with the floor. Return to the starting position.

Precautions: Keep the upper torso straight to remove stress from the lower back. Do not bounce at the bottom of the squat.

NOTE: This exercise can be performed at any selected joint angle depending on the needs of the person training.

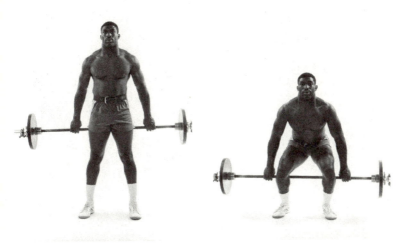

Hack Squat

Starting Position: Stand erect with the feet about shoulder width apart. The bar is placed behind the back and against the thighs. Grasp the bar with an overhand grip, and keep the head up and the back straight.

Action: Lower the body until the thighs are parallel with the floor. Return to the starting position.

Precautions: Keep the upper torso straight to remove stress from the lower back. Do not bounce at the bottom of the squat.

NOTE: This exercise can be performed at any selected joint angle depending on the needs of the person training.

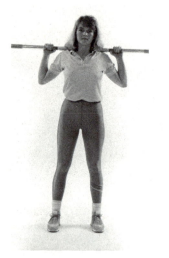
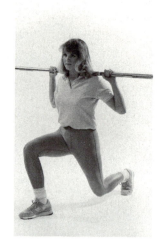

Lunge Squat

Starting Position: Stand erect with the feet about shoulder width apart. Place the bar behind the neck and across the shoulders. Keep the head up and the back straight.

Action: Step forward with the right leg and lower the body until the left knee is about twelve inches from the floor. Return to the starting position. Repeat the same action with the left leg, and return to the starting position.

Precautions: Keep the back straight and the head up during the movement. Do not bounce at the bottom part of the exercise.

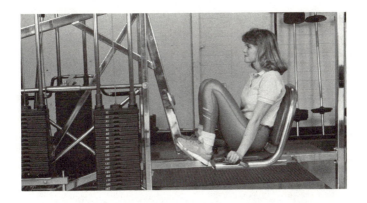

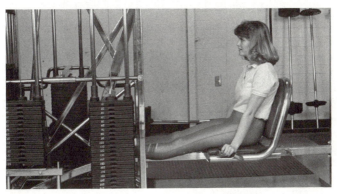

Leg Press

Starting Position: Take a seat in the machine, and grasp the handles on both sides of the seat with the feet on the pedals. Keep the back straight.

Action: Push forward until the legs are fully extended. Return to the starting position.

Precautions: Do not use any unnecessary body motion to aid in the movement.

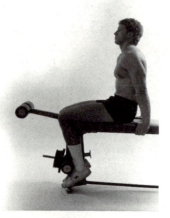 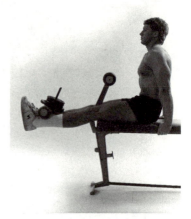

Leg Extension

Starting Position: Sit on the edge of the seat and place your feet be-hind the pads of the machine. Support the body by grasping the sides of the bench. Keep the back straight.

Action: Fully extend the legs to a locked position. Return to the starting position.

Precautions: Do not jerk the weight or use any unnecessary body motion in the movement.

NOTE: It is possible to isolate the leg muscles by doing single leg extensions.

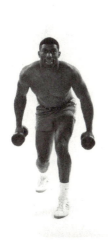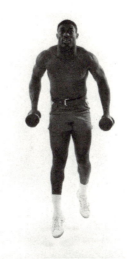

Dumbbell Jump Squat

Starting Position: Assume a front-back foot position, and hold the dumbbells with the arms fully extended. Squat down to about a 90° position.

Action: Jump upward as high as possible. Prior to returning to the starting position, switch the feet and flex the knees to absorb the downward force.

Precautions: Make sure to flex the ankles, knees, and hips when landing to reduce the downward shock.

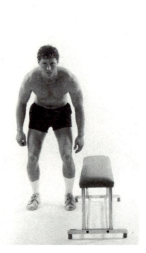 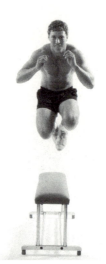

Bench Jump

Starting Position: Stand erect with the body sideways to the bench.

Action: Flex the knees and jump sideways over the bench. Touch this side and return to the starting side.

Precautions: Use the arms to aid in the jump to increase height. Make sure to flex the ankles, knees, and hips when landing to reduce the downward shock.

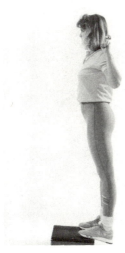 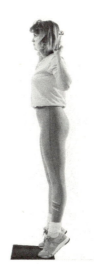

Standing Heel Raise

Starting Position: Stand erect with the feet about eight inches apart. Place the bar behind the neck and across the shoulders. Keep the head up and the back straight. Put the balls of the feet on a four-inch wooden board, and allow the heels to lower as far as possible.

Action: Raise the body as high as possible. Return to the starting position.

Precautions: Keep the body erect, and do the exercise slowly to maintain balance.

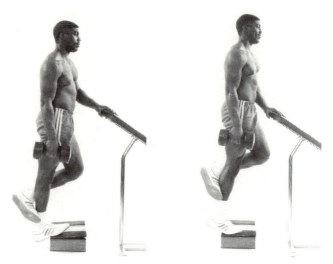

Single-Heel Raise

Starting Position: Place the right foot on a four-inch board, and allow the heel to lower as far as possible. Hold a dumbbell in the right hand with the arm extended. Keep the body erect and balanced by holding on to a support with the left hand.

Action: Raise the body as high as possible. Return to the starting position. When the repetitions for the right leg have been completed, switch to the left leg.

Precautions: Keep the body erect, and do the exercise slowly to maintain balance.

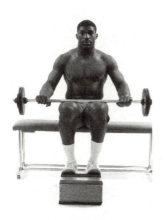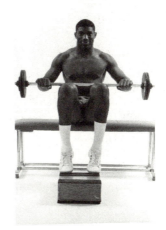

Sitting Heel Raise

Starting Position: Take a seated position on the bench. Place the bar across the top of the thigh and support the weight with the hands. Place the balls of the feet on a four-inch wooden board, and allow the heels to lower as far as possible.

Action: Raise the heels as high as possible. Return to the starting position.

Precautions: Keep the body erect, and do not bounce at the bottom of the movement.

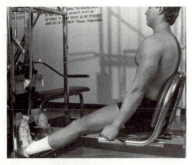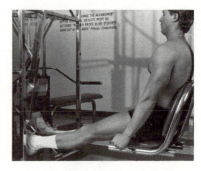

Toe Extension

Starting Position: Take a seat in the machine, and fully extend the legs. Grasp the handles on both sides of the seat, and keep the back straight. Slide the feet off the pedals until only the balls of the feet make contact.

Action: Extend the toes as far forward as possible. Return to the starting position.

Precautions: Keep the legs straight, and do the exercise slowly.

NOTE: To change the calf development it is possible to use different toe placements on the pedals as shown in the pictures.

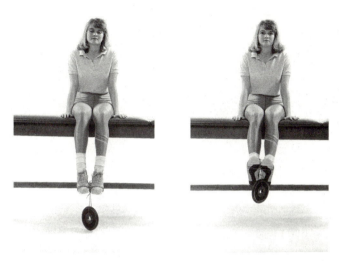

Toe Raise

Starting Position: Sit on the edge of a table with the lower legs hanging over the side. Grasp the side of the table with the hands to maintain balance. Attach a weight to the toes of the foot with a strap or rope.

Action: Lift the toes upward toward the shins as far as possible. Return to the starting position.

Precautions: Isolate the movement of the front part of the foot, and do the exercise slowly.

NOTE: This exercise can also be performed using one foot at a time.

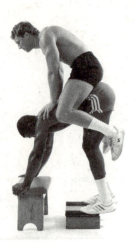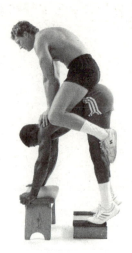

Donkey Raise

Starting Position: Bend over a bench from the waist until the upper torso is parallel to the floor. Support your body with the hands on the bench. Place the balls of the feet on a four-inch wooden board, and allow the heels to lower as far as possible. Have a partner sit astride the hips to provide resistance.

Action: Raise the body as high as possible. Return to the starting position.

Precautions: Do not use any unnecessary motion in the movement. Have the partner sit back as far as possible because this will provide more resistance in the exercise.

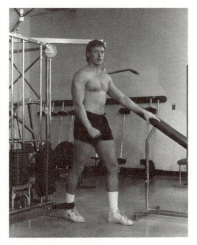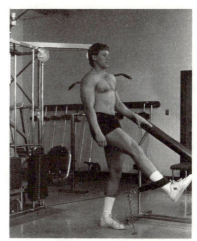

Front Leg Kick

Starting Position: Stand erect with the right leg attached to pulley from the machine. Maintain balance by holding on to a support. The right foot is approximately sixteen inches behind the left foot.

Action: Extend the right leg forward and as high as possible. Return to starting position. When the repetitions for the right leg have been completed, switch to the left leg.

Precautions: Keep the leg straight at all times, and do not bend the knee. Do the exercise slowly to maintain balance.

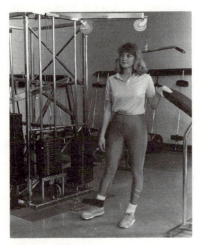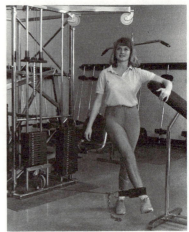

Side Leg Kick

Starting Position: Stand erect and sideways to the machine with the right leg attached to the pulley. Maintain balance by holding on to a support. The right leg is crossed over the left leg away from the machine as far as possible.

Action: Extend the right leg outward as far as possible. Return to the starting position. When the repetitions for the right leg have been completed, switch to the left.

Precautions: Keep the leg straight at all times, and do not bend the knee. Do the exercise slowly to maintain balance.

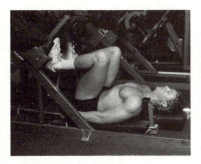 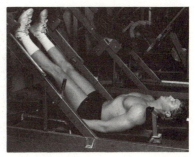

Vertical Leg Press

Starting Position: Lie flat on the back with the legs bent and the feet against the bar. The hips should be directly beneath the feet.

Action: Push the bar upward until the legs are fully extended. Return to the starting position.

Precautions: Since the resistance on this exercise has a tendency to cause the pressure in the chest cavity to increase, the lifter should keep the mouth open during the movement.

NOTE: This exercise can be modified so that the calf muscles can be trained by extending the front of the foot while the legs are extended.

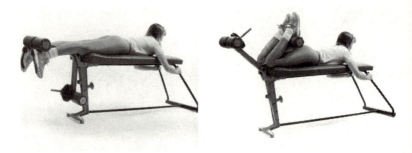

Leg Curl

Starting Position: Lie face downward on the bench with the legs extended and the backs of the feet against the pads. Grasp the sides of the bench to maintain balance.

Action: Lift the feet upward until the pads touch the buttocks. Return to the starting position.

Precautions: Movement should be entirely in the knee joint. Avoid unnecessary jerking or body movement.

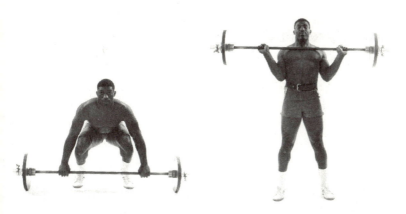

Power Clean

Starting Position: Place the feet about shoulder width apart, and allow the shins to touch the bar. Bend down and grasp the bar with an overhand grip with the hands about shoulder width on the bar. Bend the knee until the hips are slightly lower than the knees. Keep the head up and the arms fully extended.

Action: Straighten the legs to lift the weight. Keep the arms extended. Push forward with the hips as the legs extend upward. As the body starts to become erect, pull upward with the arms and bend the elbows to lift the weight to the shoulders. Move the elbows under the bar, and support the bar across the chest at the base of the neck. Reverse the procedure, and return to the starting position.

Precautions: Be sure you use an explosive movement in this exercise. Start with a light weight and practice the technique before using heavy weights.

Strength Training for Athletes

Anyone who wishes to improve athletic performance can do so by utilizing strength training. As indicated in Chapter One, to increase power, the rate of doing work, one must increase either strength or speed or, if possible, both of these factors. Since all athletic contests are time related, a person who can increase work output for a given time frame will be more successful.

Research concerning speed and strength indicates a high correlation between strength levels and speed. In the past there were some misconceptions that weight training would reduce flexibility or cause a person to be "muscle-bound" and slow. The research refutes this myth and indicates instead that by using weight training, through a full range of motion, athletes actually improve their flexibility and speed of movement.

The advantage of increased strength is important to both male and female athletes. Both can engage in a strength development program to increase their efficiency in any sport.

To design training programs utilizing weight training, it is necessary to be familiar with the basic anatomy and various movements of the human body. Figure 6.1 contains a diagram of the muscles and definitions of the muscle actions. Table 6.1 lists the name of the muscle, the action of the muscle, and the sport in which the muscle is used. By using this information, the coach or athlete can analyze a sport to determine the most important movements and the muscles involved. For example, muscle No. 26, the trapezius, tilts the head back, elevates the shoulder point, and adducts the scapula. This muscle is used in the wrestler's bridge, passing a football, cleaning a barbell, the breast stroke, archery, and batting.

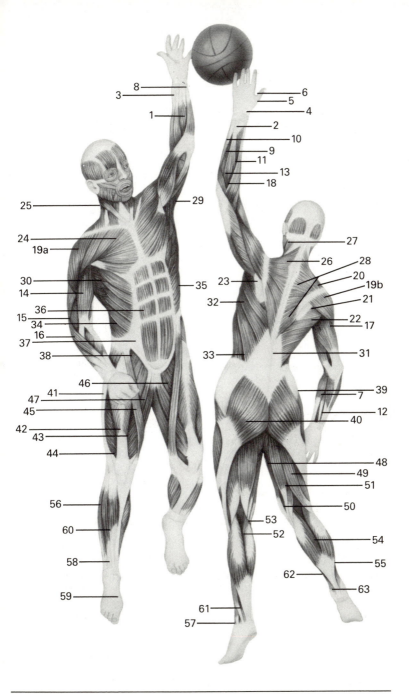

Figure 6.1   Major Human Muscles

Table 6.1 Muscle Action and Sport Use

Muscle	Primary Action Numbers in ( ) indicate muscles that assist	Sport In which greatest resistance is encountered
1. Flexor digitorum-profundus	Flexes fingers	Any sport in which one grasps an opponent, partner, or equipment, such as wrestling, hand-to-hand balancing, tennis, horizontal bar, ball bat, etc.
2. Extensor digitorum	Extends fingers	
3. Flexor pollicis longus	Flexes thumb	
4. Extensor pollicis longus	Extends thumb	
5. Abductor pollicis longus	Abducts thumb	
6. Adductor pollicis longus	Adducts and flexes thumb	
7. Flexor carpi radialis	Flexes wrist palmward (8), abducts hand (9)	Tennis, throwing a baseball, passing a football, handball, ring work, two-handed pass in basketball, batting, golf swing
8. Flexor carpi ulnaris	Flexes wrist palmward (7), adducts hand (10)	
9. Extensor carpi radialis longus and brevis	Extends wrist (10), abducts hand (7)	Backhand stroke in tennis and badminton, Olympic weight lifting, bait and fly casting
10. Extensor carpi ulnaris	Extends wrist (9), adducts hand (8)	
11. Pronator teres	Pronates forearm	Tennis forehand, shot put, throwing a punch, throwing a baseball, passing a football
12. Pronator quadratus		
13. Supinator	Supinates forearm (16)	Throwing a curve ball, batting, fencing thrust
14. Biceps brachii	Flexes forearm (16)	Ring work, rope climb, archery, pole vaulting, wrestling, back stroke in swimming
15. Brachialis		
16. Brachioradialis	Flexes forearm, supinates forearm	Rowing, cleaning a barbell, rope climb

Muscle	Primary Action Numbers in ( ) indicate muscles that assist	Sport In which greatest resistance is encountered
17. Triceps brachii 18. Anconeus	Extends forearm	Breast stroke, shot put, parallel bar work, vaulting, hand shivers in football, hand balancing, batting, pole vaulting, fencing thrust, passing, boxing

19. Deltoid
    Anterior fibers
    Posterior fibers
20. Supraspinatus
21. Infraspinatus
22. Teres Minor
	Abducts humerus (20)
	Flexes humerus
	Extends humerus
	Abducts humerus (19)
	Rotates humerus laterally
		Hand balancing, canoeing, shot put, pole vaulting, tennis, archery, batting, fencing thrust, passing a football, tackling, breast stroke, back and crawl strokes, golf swing, handball

23. Teres major	Adducts, extends, and rotates humerus medially (32)	Rope climb, canoe racing, ring work, rowing, batting, crawl, back, breast and butterfly strokes, pole vaulting, golf
24. Pectoralis major	Adducts, flexes, and rotates humerus	Tackling, crawl and back strokes, tennis, passing a football, throwing a baseball, javelin, pole vaulting, wrestling, shot put, discus throw, straight-arm lever position in gymnastics, punching
25. Sternocleido-mastoid	Flexes and laterally flexes neck, rotates head (27)	Crawl stroke, tucking chin in wrestling, football, boxing, distance running (breathing)
26. Trapezius	Bends head laterally toward shoulder	Wrestler's bridge

Muscle	Primary Action Numbers in ( ) indicate muscles that assist	Sport In which greatest resistance is encountered
	Elevates shoulder	Passing a football, cleaning a barbell, breast stroke
	Adducts scapula	Archery, batting, breast stroke
27. Splenius cervicis/ capitus	Extends head back Extends head (26) Rotates head	
28. Major and minor rhomboids, levator scapulae	Adducts and rotates scapula medially, depresses shoulder	Tennis backhand, batting, back and breast stroke
29. Subscapularis	Rotates humerus medially (24), stabilizes humerus in glenoid cavity to prevent displacement	Tackling, crawl and back strokes, tennis, passing a football, throwing a baseball, javelin, pole vaulting, wrestling, shot put, discus throw, straight-arm level position in gymnastics
30. Serratus anterior	Abducts scapula	Shot put, discus throw, tennis, archery, tackling, crawl stroke, passing a basketball, passing a football, punching
31. Erector spinae	Extends vertebral column	Discus and hammer throw, batting, golf swing, racing start in swimming, diving and tumbling, rowing, blocking in football
32. Latissimus dorsi	Adducts, extends, and rotates humerus medially; depresses shoulder	Rope climb, canoe racing, ring work, rowing, batting, crawl, back, breast, and butterfly strokes, pole vaulting, golf swing

Muscle	Primary Action Numbers in ( ) indicate muscles that assist	Sport In which greatest resistance is encountered
33. Quadratus lumborum	Flexes vertebral column, flexes vertebral column laterally	The importance of this group in all sports, posture, and general fitness and appearance cannot be overstated
34. External abdominal oblique	Flexes and rotates vertebral column	
35. Internal abdominal oblique		
36. Rectus abdominus	Flexes vertebral column (33)	
37. Transverse abdominus	Compresses abdomen	
38. Iliopsoas, pectineus	Flexes femur (42)	Running, hurdling, pole vaulting, kicking a football, line play, flutter kick, pike and tuck positions in diving and tumbling
39. Gluteus medius	Abducts femur, rotates femur medially	Hurdling, fencing, frog kick, shot put, running, line play, skating
40. Gluteus maximus	Extends femur, rotates femur laterally	Skiing, shot put, running, quick starts in track, all jumping and skipping, line play, skating, swimming start, changing directions while running
41. Tensor fasciae	Flexes, abducts and rotates femur medially	
42. Rectus femoris	Extends lower leg (43, 44), flexes femur	Skiing, skating, quick starts, all jumping, kick in football or soccer, flutter kick, frog kick, water skiing, diving, trampoline and tumbling, bicycling, catching in baseball
43. Vastus medialis	Extends lower leg	
44. Vastus lateralis		
45. Sartorius	Flexes lower leg, flexes femur, rotates femur laterally	

Muscle	Primary Action Numbers in ( ) indicate muscles that assist	Sport In which greatest resistance is encountered
46. Adductor magnus	Adducts femur (48)	Skiing, skating, frog kick, broken field running, bareback horseback riding
47. Adductor longus		
48. Gracilis	Adducts femur, flexes lower leg	
49. Biceps femoris	Flexes lower leg, rotates lower leg laterally (53, 54); extends femur (48, 50, 51)	Skiing, skating, quick starts in track and swimming, hurdling line play, all jumping
50. Semimembranosus	Flexes lower leg, rotates lower leg medially (52)	
51. Semitendinosus	Extends femur	
52. Popliteus	Flexes lower leg, rotates lower leg medially	
53. Plantaris	Plantar flexes foot (when knee is almost straight)	Quick starts in track, swimming, basketball, football, skating, all jumping, skiing
54. Gastrocnemius	Flexes lower leg	
55. Soleus	Plantar flexes foot	
56. Peroneus longus	Plantar flexes and everts foot	Changing directions while running, skating, skiing, running, all jumping, racing starts, skating turns
57. Peroneus brevis		
58. Extensor digitorum	Extends the four smaller toes	
59. Extensor hallicus	Extends the big toe	
60. Tibialis anterior	Dorsiflexes and inverts foot	
61. Tibialis posterior	Plantar flexes and inverts foot	
62. Flexor digitorum longus	Flexes the four smaller toes	
63. Flexor hallicus longus	Flexes the big toe	

Adapted from Muscle Action Chart by Cramer Products, Inc. Reprinted by permission of Cramer Products, Inc., P.O. Box 1001, Gardner KS 66030.

STRENGTH TRAINING

Flex: bend at a joint, decreasing angle
Extend: straighten at a joint
Adduct: move toward midline of body
Abduct: move away from midline
Rotate: move part around an axis
Prone: face downward
Supine: face upward
Pronate: rotate forearm to palms-down
Supinate: rotate forearm to palms-up
Invert: turn sole of foot inward
Evert: turn sole of foot inward
Evert: turn sole of foot outward
Elevate: raise a part against gravity
Depress: lower a part, yielding to gravity
Lateral: located toward the outer side
Medial: located toward the middle

Sport Training Worksheet

Name _____

Exercise	Sets	Reps	Resistance

Table 6.2 Weight Training Exercises for Specific Sports

	Arm curl	Back raise	Bench flys	Bench jump	Bench press	Bent-arm pullover	Bent-over lateral raise	Bent-over rowing	Curl-up	Dead lift	Dip	Dumbbell bent-over rowing	Dumbbell curl	Heel raise
Archery	X		X		X		X		X				X	
Badminton			X			X								
Baseball					X		X		X		X		X	
Basketball	X			X					X		X			
Bicycling					X				X					
Bowling	X	X			X				X					X
Boxing		X			X			X						
Canoeing						X	X	X						
Climbing	X				X		X		X		X			
Crew	X	X			X		X					X		
Diving					X				X					
Fencing					X				X					
Field hockey	X		X		X				X					X
Football	X				X	X				X	X		X	
Golf	X				X		X							
Handball		X			X				X					
Hockey	X	X			X				X		X			
Martial arts	X	X			X		X		X					X

STRENGTH TRAINING

Incline bench press	Lat-pulldown	Leg curl	Leg extension	Leg press	Neck exercise	Overhead press	Power clean	Seated heel raise	Seated rowing	Side lateral raise	Single-heel raise	Squat	Toe extension	Triceps extension	Twists	Upright rowing	Wrist curls
	■	■		■								■	■	■	■	■	■
	■	■	■									■	■		■	■	
	■											■	■	■		■	■
	■		■								■	■	■			■	■
	■															■	
	■		■			■				■		■	■			■	■
■	■									■		■	■	■			
■	■	■				■						■					■
■	■	■								■		■					■
	■					■				■		■					
■								■		■		■	■	■		■	
■									■		■		■		■		■
■	■	■		■		■			■		■		■	■		■	■
	■	■									■		■	■	■	■	■
	■	■	■								■		■	■		■	■
■	■										■		■	■	■	■	■
	■	■				■					■	■	■	■		■	

	Arm curl	Back raise	Bench flys	Bench jump	Bench press	Bent-arm pullover	Bent-over lateral raise	Bent-over rowing	Curl-up	Dead lift	Dip	Dumbbell bent-over rowing	Dumbbell curl	Heel raise
Racquetball		■			■		■		■		■			
Rugby	■	■			■				■				■	■
Skating		■							■					
Skiing	■	■												
Soccer					■	■								
Softball	■		■			■	■	■	■			■	■	■
Squash	■	■			■	■	■	■	■					
Swimming		■			■	■		■	■					
Tennis	■	■	■		■		■		■				■	■
Track-distance	■	■					■		■					
Track-sprints		■			■				■					
Field events	■	■	■		■				■			■		
Volleyball					■								■	■
Water Polo	■				■				■				■	■
Wrestling	■	■			■	■			■			■		

Incline bench press	Lat-pulldown	Leg curl	Leg extension	Leg press	Neck exercise	Overhead press	Power clean	Seated heel raise	Seated rowing	Side lateral raise	Single-heel raise	Squat	Toe extension	Triceps extension	Twists	Upright rowing	Wrist curls
	■	■						■		■		■	■	■	■	■	
■	■	■	■	■	■	■			■			■	■		■	■	
	■	■									■	■		■	■	■	
	■	■	■						■		■	■	■	■	■		
	■	■							■		■	■	■	■	■	■	
	■					■					■	■	■	■	■	■	■
	■								■		■	■	■		■	■	■
	■	■							■			■	■	■	■	■	■
	■	■		■					■		■	■	■	■	■	■	■
	■	■			■						■	■	■	■	■	■	
	■	■	■	■					■		■	■	■	■	■	■	
■	■	■	■				■				■	■	■	■	■	■	■
	■	■				■			■			■	■		■	■	
	■	■		■	■				■		■	■	■		■	■	■

Table 5.1 in Chapter 5 has a list of exercises for selected body parts. By referring to Figure 6.1, which describes the location of the various muscles, we find that the trapezius is located in the back. One might choose the lat-pulldown or pull-up from Table 5.1 as an exercise to increase the strength of the trapezius.

Table 6.2 lists various sports and weight training exercises that should be considered to increase the strength of the muscles used in the sport. To determine the number of repetitions, consider whether the sport requires an emphasis on strength or on muscular endurance. As indicated in Chapter 2, the rule to follow is:

Increased strength = decrease the repetitions, increase the resistance

Increased endurance = increase the repetitions, decrease the resistance

Following is an example of how the information in Tables 6.1 and 6.2 can be used to write an off-season strength program for football. This is a program that has been followed for past years by the highly successful Brigham Young University football program, under the direction of the outstanding conditioning coach, Dr. Chuck Stiggins.

BYU FOOTBALL OFF-SEASON STRENGTH TRAINING PROGRAM

Note: The major factor behind the number of repetitions completed in each set is that the last repetition must be a total maximum effort.

Warm-up: Start each exercise with a warm-up set using a resistance that is approximately 40 percent of your 1 RM for 8–10 repetitions.

Monday

Bench press	Sets	1-2-3-4
	Repetitions	6-5-4-3 RM
Incline bench press (dumbbells, if possible)	Sets	1-2-3
	Repetitions	6-5-4 RM
Weighted dips	2 sets of 8 RM	
Triceps extension	2 sets of 8 RM	
Seated overhead press	Sets	1-2-3
	Repetitions	6-5-4 RM

Arm curls	Sets	1-2-3
	Repetitions	8-6-6 RM
Squats	Sets	1-2-3-4-5
	Repetitions	6-5-5-4-3 RM
Leg curls	Sets	1-2-3-4
	Repetitions	8-6-6-6 RM
Curl-ups	3 sets of 25 repetitions	
Neck exercise	3 sets of 10 repetitions	

The weight resistance for the following exercises will be at 70 percent of the 1RM and no higher.

Power cleans	Sets	1-2-3
	Repetitions	8-6-6 RM
Dead lifts	Sets	1-2-3
	Repetitions	8-6-6 RM

Wednesday

Incline press	3 sets of 8 RM
Triceps extension	3 sets of 8 RM
Lat-pulldown	3 sets of 8 RM
Shrugs	3 sets of 8 RM
Leg extensions	3 sets of 8 RM
Leg curls	3 sets of 8 RM
Curl-ups	3 sets of 25 repetitions
Neck exercise	3 sets of 10 repetitions

Friday

Bench press	Sets	1-2-3-4
	Repetitions	5-4-4-3 RM
Incline bench press	Sets	1-2-3
	Repetitions	6-5-4 RM
Weighted dips	2 sets of 8 RM	
Triceps extension	2 sets of 8 RM	
Seated overhead press	Sets	1-2-3
	Repetitions	6-5-4 RM
Arm curls	Sets	1-2-3
	Repetitions	8-6-6 RM
Squats	Sets	1-2-3
	Repetitions	6-5-5 RM
Leg curls	Sets	1-2-3
	Repetitions	8-6-6 RM
Curl-ups	3 sets of 25 repetitions	
Neck exercise	3 sets of 10 repetitions	

Strength Training for Athletes

By using the information contained in this chapter, an athlete or coach can devise individualized strength training programs for any sport.

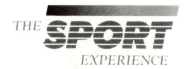

THE **SPORT** EXPERIENCE

Write an individualized strength training program for your selected sport by using the suggested exercises listed in Table 6.2, "Weight Training Exercises for Specific Sports," and record your workout program on the Sport Training Worksheet.

Remember:

1. If you want to emphasize increased strength, you decrease the number of repetitions and increase the resistance.
2. If you want to emphasize increased muscle endurance, you increase the number of repetitions and decrease the resistance.

STRENGTH TRAINING

Physique Training and Bodybuilding

Bodybuilder is defined as a person who uses srength training to obtain a more muscular physique. When it is defined this way, nearly all people who lift weights can be classified as bodybuilders. As indicated before, the author has found that the majority of men and women that enroll in beginning weight training classes do so because of a desire to "look better," or, in other words, they wish to be "bodybuilders."

By using the training programs explained previously, it is possible to develop the different muscles of the body and bring about a more muscular physique.

Another group of individuals who have a great desire to affect the muscular system of the body are classified as physique athletes. The elite athletes in this group would be those who earn Mr. America, Mr. Universe, or Mr. Olympia titles. This would also include females who compete for simlar titles such as Miss America and Miss Universe.

Most physique contests are judged on the following basis:

1. *Symmetry:* the overall balance of development of the various body parts and muscle groups.
2. *Muscularity:* how well a muscle is developed in regard to size, definition, and hardness.
3. *Presentation:* personal grooming, posing ability, and how individuals project themselves.

It is impossible for people to see themselves as they really are even when using a mirror. We many times view ourselves quite differently than what is reflected. To record changes and understand more about your body, you should measure the various body parts at the start of a training program and take periodic measurements to determine how the training is affecting the body size.

Another method to determine how the body looks is to have a series of photographs taken of yourself in a swimsuit. Have photos taken of the front, side, and back, with the body in a relaxed position and then with the muscles flexed. This will give information that can be used later, after you have been training, to compare with the changes that take place. It is true that "a picture is worth a thousand words."

A person's body type is determined to a great extent before birth, but through proper training, an individual can build some areas and reduce others. The purpose of this chapter will be to explain various types of physique training programs one might engage in to bring about those body changes.

There is not one best system of training because each individual is different. It is suggested that a person experiment with different systems of training and find that method which works best. A combination of the various systems may bring about the desired results and stimulate the body to make rapid gains. As suggested in the preceding paragraphs, the lifter should keep accurate records of how the body responded to the different methods of training. By comparing the progress made, it now becomes easier to select the most beneficial training regimen.

SYSTEMS OF TRAINING

Set System.   The set system is the most popular type of training to develop strength. In this system the person does an exercise for a given number of repetitions, or set, then rests, and then performs another set. A variation of this system is referred to as *supersets,* in which an exercise set for a particular muscle group is followed immediately by an exercise set for the antagonist muscle. An example of this training system would be to do a set of arm curls for the biceps and then do a set of triceps extensions for the triceps. This combination would be one superset.

Another variation of this type of training is known as the "super multiple set system." In this training system the lifter completes all of the sets for a given muscle group and then follows this exercise with the same number of sets for the antagonist muscle group.

Split Routine.   In bodybuilding the idea is to exercise every major muscle group in the body, and this requires a great amount of time and work. To obtain the maximum development, the major body parts are split into groups, and the lifter works out six days a week but exercises the selected body parts on alternate days. For example, the arms, legs and midsection might be exercised on Monday, Wednesday, and Friday, and the chest, shoulders, and back would be exercised on Tuesday, Thursday, and Saturday. This system is one of the most popular types of training used by bodybuilders. Often this training program incorporates supersets.

A variation of the split-routine system is known as the *blitz method*. This is often utilized when the bodybuilder is preparing for a contest and wishes to obtain the maximum size and muscle definition so important in competition. In this system a person would perform all the arm exercises one day, the next day engage in just chest exercises, the legs on the next day, and follow each day with another body part. This is a very strenuous and tiring method of training and is usually recommended only for a few weeks at a time.

Burns.   Some bodybuilders include sets of rapid half-contractions, or "burns," in their workout. The reason is to produce a burning sensation in the muscle, which is thought to be due to the forcing of blood into the muscle area to produce the so-called *muscle pump.* The result that the lifter is trying to achieve is a greater increase in the size of the musculature.

Forced Reps. The forced-reps method of training requires the use of a partner who assists the lifter so that more repetitions with greater resistance can be accomplished. The partner can push the individual far beyond the normal point of fatigue, the hoped-for result being more strength and muscle-building stimulation. For example, an individual might do ten repetitions on the lat-pulldown without assistance. When the person reaches the normal point of fatigue on the tenth repetition, the partner would assist the lifter through the sticking point for three to five more "forced reps."

Pre-exhaustion.   Most exercises in strength training are accomplished by a large muscle group working in conjunction with a smaller muscle group. For example, the back muscles work with the biceps of the arm in pull-ups. The small muscle may fatigue before the large muscle group, and as a result, the large muscle group does not receive the optimum resistance to bring about physiological changes, such as an increase in size.

The pre-exhaustion system is based on the idea of doing a preliminary isolation exercise to overload the large muscle group before doing the exercise that uses both the large and small muscle groups together. This technique theoretically would then fatigue the stronger group to make it weaker than the smaller muscle group, and thus the lifter could now push the basic combination exercise to a point where both muscle groups would develop.

Pyramid System. This type of training consists of adding weight until the lifter can only complete one repetition. For example, a person may start doing the bench press with a set of 10 RM. Then add enough weight to do 9 RM, then 8 RM, and so on until the final set would consist of 1 RM.

In the first type of pyramid the lifter went from light to heavy resistance. There is another pyramid system where one goes from heavy to light resistance. After a warm-up set the lifter does a set of 1–2 RM, removes, for example, five pounds, and does the maximum number of repetitions and continues to do this until only the weight of the bar or a small resistance remains.

In the following section is a training program that was utilized by a student of the author who placed first in the Mr. Collegiate USA contest.

WEIGHT TRAINING FOR BODYBUILDERS

Basic Concepts

1. Every major muscle group in the body is exercised.
2. The musculature is worked as thoroughly as possible (achieving a "pumped" feeling).
3. Every set is preceded by a rest period of no more than 90 seconds.
4. Every repetition is performed in the strictest form.
5. The emphasis in bodybuilding is placed on doing the exercise movement correctly rather than trying to lift as much weight as possible.
6. A set of high repetitions begins each initial exercise per major muscle group, and as the resistance increases the repetitions decrease.

Split Routine Program to be Followed Six Days a Week

Work the following every day:

1. Abdominals
2. Chest: Heavy one day, reps the next
   a. Heavy: Dumbbell bench press; bench press to neck; bench flys
   b. Reps: Bent-arm pullovers
3. Calves: Heavy one day, reps the next
   a. Heavy: Toe extensions, single-heel raises
   b. Reps: Toe extensions

First Day

Roman chair curl-ups	3 sets of 75 reps, 3 sets of 80 reps
V-sits	6 sets of 45 reps
Hanging knee-ups	6 sets of 25 reps
Arm curls	1 set of 10 reps, 1 set of 8 reps, 3 sets of 6 reps
Standing dumbbell curls	5 sets of 8 reps
Incline dumbbell curls	5 sets of 8 reps
Triceps pressdowns	4 sets of 8 reps, 1 set of 6 reps
Lying barbell triceps extensions	1 set of 10 reps, 4 sets of 8 reps
Seated dumbbell triceps extensions	2 sets of 10 reps, 2 sets of 8 reps, 1 set of 6 reps
Front squats	1 set of 20 reps, 1 set of 16 reps, 1 set of 12 reps, 1 set of 10 reps
Lunge squats	1 set of 12 reps, 3 sets of 10 reps
Leg extensions	2 sets of 25 reps, 1 set of 16 reps, 1 set of 12 reps
Leg curls	4 sets of 12 reps, 1 set of 20 reps
Toe extensions	5 sets of 20 reps, 3 sets of 25 reps
Single-heel raises	5 sets of 14 reps, 2 sets of 50 reps
Bent-arm pullovers	6 sets of 8 reps

Second Day

Roman chair curl-ups	3 sets of 75 reps, 3 sets of 80 reps
V-sits	6 sets of 45 reps
Hanging knee-ups	6 sets of 25 reps *(see p. 128)*

(see p. 128)

Physique Training and Bodybuilding

Dumbbell bench press	1 set of 10 reps, 3 sets of 8 reps, 1 set of 6 reps
Bench press to neck	1 set of 12 reps, 1 set of 10 reps, 2 sets of 8 reps, 1 set of 6 reps
Decline press	1 set of 10 reps, 1 set of 8 reps, 3 sets of 6 reps
Bench flys	2 sets of 10 reps, 1 set of 8 reps, 2 sets of 6 reps
Close grip lat-pulldown	2 sets of 10 reps, 2 sets of 9 reps
Regular grip lat-pulldown	1 set of 10 reps, 2 sets of 9 reps, 1 set of 7 reps
Seated rowing	3 sets of 10 reps, 1 set of 9 reps
Seated behind-neck press	2 sets of 7 reps, 2 sets of 6 reps
Seated dumbbell press	5 sets of 12 reps
Upright rowing	1 set of 10 reps, 4 sets of 9 reps
Side lateral raises	5 sets of 8 reps
Toe extensions	6 sets of 25 reps

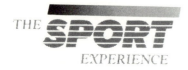

THE SPORT EXPERIENCE

Write a bodybuilding training program for yourself using the Bodybuilding Worksheet.

Remember:

1. Before starting your bodybuilding program, take all your body measurements using the Body Measurement Chart so that you can plot your progress as you train.
2. If possible, take some photographs of yourself before starting your training program, and then you will be able to compare how you look at various stages of your training program.
3. Work every major muscle group in your body.
4. Experiment with various bodybuilding systems of training during your program to determine which works best for you.

Bodybuilding Training Worksheet

Name _____

Body Part	Exercise	Sets	Reps	Resistance
Chest				
Midsection				
Triceps				
Legs				
Shoulders				
Neck				
Biceps				
Back				

Physique Training and Bodybuilding

Appendix A
Periodicals on Strength Development

1. *Health and Strength.* Health and Strength Publishing Company, Ltd., Halton House, 20-23 Holborn, London E.C.1, United Kingdom.
2. *Iron Man.* Iron Man Publishing Company, 512 Black Hills Avenue, Alliance, Nebraska 69301.
3. *Muscle and Fitness.* Muscle Builder Publications, Inc., 2110 Erwin Street, Woodland Hills, California 91364.
4. *Muscle Mag International.* Health Culture Subscription Department, 270 Rutherford Road South, Bramptom, Ontario, Canada L6W 3K7.
5. *Muscle Training Illustrated.* Muscle Man, Inc., 1664 Utica Avenue, Brooklyn, New York 11234.
6. *Muscular Development.* Muscular Development, P.O. Box 1707, York, Pennsylvania 17405.
7. *National Strength and Conditioning Association Journal.* National Strength and Conditioning Association, P.O. Box 81410, Lincoln, Nebraska 68501.
8. *Powerman.* Powerman Magazine, P.O. Box 3005, Erie, Pennsylvania 16508.
9. *Strength and Health.* Strength and Health, P.O. Box 1707, York, Pennsylvania 17405.

Body Measurement Chart

Name _____ Age _____

Date											
Body Weight											
Neck											
Shoulders											
Chest	Relaxed										
	Flexed										
Upper Arm Relaxed	Right										
	Left										
Flexed	Right										
	Left										
Forearm Relaxed	Right										
	Left										
Flexed	Right										
	Left										
Waist											
Hips											
Thigh Relaxed	Right										
	Left										
Flexed	Right										
	Left										
Calf Relaxed	Right										
	Left										
Flexed	Right										
	Left										
Other Body Parts											

Appendix C
Strength Training Record

Name _____   Age _____

Date					
Exercise	Wt Reps	Wt Reps	Wt Reps	Wt Reps	Wt Reps

Wt Reps	Wt Reps	Wt Reps	Wt Reps	Wt Reps	Wt Reps

Appendix C Strength Training Record

Appendix D
Bibliography

Allsen, Philip E. *Conditioning and Physical Fitness: Current Answers to Relevant Questions.* William C. Brown Company Publishers, Dubuque, Iowa, 1978.

Allsen, Philip E., Joyce M. Harrison, and Barbara Vance. *Fitness for Life: An Individualized Approach,* William C. Brown Company Publishers, Dubuque, Iowa, 1984.

American College of Sports Medicine. "Position Statement on the Use and Abuse of Anabolic-Androgenic Steroids in Sports." *Medicine and Science in Sports,* 9(1977):xi–xiii.

Hatfield, Frederick C., and March Krotee. *Personalized Weight Training for Fitness and Athletics.* Kendall-Hunt Publishing Company, Dubuque, Iowa, 1984.

O'Shea, John P. *Scientific Principles and Methods of Strength Fitness.* Addison-Wesley Publishing Company, Reading, Massachusetts, 1976.

Rasch, Philip J. *Weight Training.* William C. Brown Company Publishers, Dubuque, Iowa, 1982.

Riley, Daniel P. *Strength Training by the Experts.* Leisure Press, West Point, New York, 1977.

Snyder, George, and Rick Wayne. *3 More Reps,* Olympus Health and Recreation, Inc., Warrington, Pennsylvania, 1978.

Sprague, Ken. *The Gold's Gym Book of Strength Training.* J. P. Tracher, Inc., Los Angeles, California, 1979.

Tufen, Rich, Clancy Moore, and Virgil Knight. *Weight Training for Everyone.* Hunter Publishing Company, Winston-Salem, North Carolina, 1982.

Westcott, Wayne L. *Strength Fitness: Physiological Principles and Training Techniques.* Allyn and Bacon, Inc., Boston, Massachusetts, 1982.

Williams, Melvin H. *Nutrition for Fitness and Sport.* William C. Brown Company Publishers, Dubuque, Iowa, 1983.

Index

9852